Autism, Family & You

Ian Hale, Ph.D.

Foreword by Newton Lee
Afterword by Chloe Estelle

In memory of Dr. Harold (Hackie) Reitman

Autism, Family & You
by Ian Hale, Ph.D.

ISBN 979-8-9853763-1-9

Cover Photo: Chloe Estelle & Benji by Annette Lombardi.
Other images in the book by "Couchtripper."

Table of Contents

Foreword

My younger brother suffered from severe level 3 autism when he was a child. He could talk but he chose not to speak up. He did not respond to sensory stimuli to the point that he did not even shed a tear when in physical pain. My parents knew nothing about autism and thought that my brother needed to be exorcised. Fortunately, he survived the ordeal against all odds, earned an MBA degree, started a business, got married, and became a father. Today he is a high-functioning autistic adult. Other success stories include Dr. Ian Hale, the author of this book, and my former student Chloe Estelle who wrote the afterword.

An April 2025 report from the U.S. Centers for Disease Control and Prevention (CDC) shows that the autism diagnosis rate has increased among children—about 1 in every 31 children in 2022, up from 1 in 36 in 2020. Secretary Robert F. Kennedy Jr. announced in April 2025 that U.S. Department of Health and Human Services (HSS) has launched a "massive testing and research effort that's going to involve hundreds of scientists from around the world." Kennedy said, "By September, we will know what has caused the autism epidemic, and we'll be able to eliminate those exposures."

Many scientists have cast doubt on the aggressive timeline, but one thing we all agree on is the urgency of tackling the autism epidemic. Dr. Ian Hale's book *Autism, Family & You* is a timely and useful must-read book for families with autistic children, teachers mentoring autistic students, as well as scholars and researchers on autism. Dr. Hale's keen insights stemmed from his personal journey in overcoming autism and his scientific analysis of the epidemic. This book shares important knowledge and wisdom to help families improve their quality of life.

Prof. Newton Lee
Institute for Education, Research, and Scholarships
Los Angeles, California

I. Hale

Reviews

"Dr. Hale has achieved with great success an in-depth knowledge of the leading viewpoints on a personal level and clinical evaluation into the definitions, findings and meanings through professional research as a top Autism Specialist in this increasingly important subject. He takes the reader into the vast and complex world of Autism in an easy-to-understand profile of the knowledge and research in these areas and the profound impact they have on people learning to cope with them in their daily lives. In society today where the population ratio has been going up for Autism in various countries worldwide and primarily in America, especially the states of California, Texas and Arizona it is vital to have a reference manual easily available to help those affected by Autism, in all its forms and stages. This book is that manual and invites the reader to come past the door to reveal what it is like to live inside the Autistic world to better educate society as a whole. Overall the book is descriptive, well-written, staggering, profound, suburb and outstanding. It merits the highest the praise. A 10+ must read."
—*The National League American Pen Women-Nashville Branch*

"Given the increasing numbers of children being diagnosed with autism, parents should welcome this book as a very valuable resource. Dr. Hale is himself a person with Asperger's who has dedicated most of his adult life to research and advocacy. His guide is easy to read and understand, full of insights. He writes from a unique, personal perspective, with warmth and understanding: Highly recommended."
—*CIS Review of Books*

"A super read: crammed with anecdotes, history, anger, practical tips, science, theory and medicine from someone who's there. Like no other book written on Autism, it takes no prisoners, unsentimental, heartfelt and at times controversial in challenging accepted positions and practice without losing its targets or sense of compassion."
—*Michael Wilkinson, Glasgow Scotland*

Preface

To be clear....it is important to frame this book into context by knowing a little of its origins. I'm a person with Autism. It is an indivisible part of who I am as an individual; it informs, goads, and limits at every moment of my life.

Technically: I have Asperger's Syndrome, with mild Autism, Dyslexia, moderate Dyscalculia and Attention Deficit Hyperactive Disorder (ADHD). To the best of my knowledge these traits have been passed down through previous generations of the family on my father's side for more than two hundred and fifty years. I have found written records: correspondence, diaries and poetry from the family archives of many forebears, including one who was put in the notorious Bethlehem Hospital in London. The original "Bedlam," a mental Asylum in mid eighteenth-century England where the public were charged an admission fee by warders to spectate on and bait the sufferings of the inmates as a form of "public entertainment", and additional income for the warders. (Hale Family Archive: Gloucester County Records Office, England).

There are times when we should ask ourselves just how far we have truthfully come in the fields of mental and indeed physical health since then. The despicable child and adult sexual and physical abuse by the English popular "entertainer," Jimmy Saville, "Diddy" and many others are prime examples. Many of those crimes were committed in public hospitals and other secure units against patients, many Autistics, mostly children and with the full knowledge both of successive governments and police forces. This is part of the grim side of Autism. It is not confined to Britain or America, but is rife across most of the world. It happens because the wider public doesn't know. To improve that lack of understanding is one fundamental reason for writing this book.

Currently there are two male and three female cousins with various Autistic statements—overall about forty percent of my generation.

In the next generation, the eldest child of one of those is identified as Asperger's, and has exceptional talents in the fields of art, sport, and Natural Sciences, another is Dyslexic, and a third is a Mathematics genius. There may be more, who knows? To paraphrase a joke, "Autism doesn't run through my family, it ambles gently around getting to know everyone personally." :)

I was blessed beyond words by the effort, support and encouragement I received from my amazing parents and Grandfather, Ewart (Also, like his older brother, Victor, Asperger's) who always backed up and believed in their "strange little boy" who grew up to become a writer, researcher, cat lover Autism advocate, Ambassador and Professor.

I am from the historic City and County of Bristol, England, a member of British Mensa, the Athenian Society and the World Academy of Medical Science. A graduate of Portsmouth, Bristol and Bath Spa Universities, my professional background is in Further and Higher Education, Special Education, and Biophysics.

Being a writer, broadcaster and practitioner specializing in Autism is one thing, but I hope that by actually being one to bring a new dimension to its understanding and implications, which is another principal reason for writing this book-only someone who lives it truly knows what it's like. This isn't an academic textbook or clinical observation- this is how it is and how it lives, good and bad.

Because of the family experience, autism was always a part of everyday, normal life for me. This understanding lends a uniquely powerful and sharply different perspective to both assessing and then providing a high quality of educational and life experience for affected people, whether children or adults-as each has their own particular viewpoint and set of needs. Autism is for life, including senior care, a fact seldom considered by social agencies. No-one "grows out" of Autism; it is not "a phase." The vulnerable child grows into a vulnerable adult at all stages of life. That is the reason why parents and carers worry so much about the future of their children and are often accused of being "fussy" or "over-protective."

The harsh truth is they are always under immense stress thinking; "what will happen to MY child when we have passed or are no longer able to protect and advocate for him/her?"

It is an alarming fact that worldwide in social services, charities and specialist units as well as Education and Medicine, all the decisions about what Autistic people need are taken by non-autistics. In the Autism community we call them NTs-Neuro-Typical and ourselves NDs-Neuro-Diverse. Surely these decisions need to be taken if not always by us, then at least in direct consultation with us. As I say, "If you don't live it, you don't know it." We know ourselves best, our right to be seen, heard and to self-determination must be respected-that is the third reason for writing this book, it's the guide I wish my family and all families had to help them positively along the way. That includes me as a kid, growing up with Autism.

Introduction

Opening the Door:

Welcome! There have been many excellent and informative books and movies about autism, Dr. Harold Reitman, founder of www.differentbrains.com, Dr. Tony Attwood, Wendy Lawson and Vera Quinn and the more famous Dr. Temple Grandin plus many more. There are also thought-provoking movies like "Rain Man" (1988), "Mercury Rising" (1998) and "My name is Khan" (2010), and most importantly, Dr. Reitman's "must see", "The square root of 2".

Additionally there are some fine websites such as www.Oasis.org and www.autismlink.com together with the websites of the famous Tomati and Karolinska Institutes in Stockholm, Sweden, the publishing house Springer Nature, and the superb www.dyslexia.org which deals minutely and accurately with a broad variety of issues in this increasingly high-profile subject. Facebook too contains specialist Autism groups, some very good, others not. It does though remain a rich source of contacts and support.

However, most of the books only examine one or two aspects of Neurodiversity as a whole, with "The Autism Spectrum" (as it is known) being one sector. Furthermore, they tend to come into one of three distinct categories. Firstly, well-meaning (sometimes) but often shallow and inaccurate "family-help" books, secondly, brilliant but impenetrably worded academic publications which concentrate on specific scientific research and theory and finally, very long books of pure symptom description. These are helpful for teachers and doctors for diagnostic purposes and education strategies, but they lack any real background information or human warmth which would place the subject more firmly in its context to enrich the everyday lives of those affected by these conditions. This book is intended to fill some of the gaps between those categories and humanize the subject, as well as to shed fresh insights upon it.

It deliberately avoids jargon and so-called "New Age Psychobabble" and seeks to demystify and rectify the problems inherent in autism by examining in clear terms the whole panorama of the subject, not just individual bits, beginning with its history and including practical advice at every level, yet without being inaccessible to a very broad readership. It unravels and demystifies medical, psychiatric and psychological terminology to reveal what autism really is and what it means to be autistic in day-to-day life and then analyzes its strengths and weaknesses in order to offer practical and constructive advice on dealing with it directly on its own terms, as it affects each individual and family.

This book is a comprehensive look at the subject, drawn from a number of avenues of thought and knowledge, including anecdotal ones, as well as a series of ideas, research and commentary gained from numerous sources around the world. It does not claim to be definitive. It is a broad, empowering guide. A complete, science-based understanding of the subject is still a long way off and any book or person who claims to have all the answers, doesn't.

It is vitally important to acknowledge as few doctors or teachers are willing to do—that autistics ("autistics" is a bit of a tricky, old-fashioned word, so from now on, we'll mostly use the more modern "Autists") are people first and patients who happen to have a form or forms of autism second. While accepting that resources were already limited before the economic crises of today, what is unacceptable is that the existing funding is being cut once again- and solely because autistics are a minority voter group-only around 1.2% of any given population—a cowardly form of social targeting and victimization.

A further aim of this guide is to inform and by doing so empower all those whose lives are touched by autism to speak out against the discrimination, ignorance, abandonment and harassment that Autists routinely suffer at the hands of largely uncaring or uninformed authority and institutions around the world on a twenty-four-hour basis.

I. Hale

Chapter 1: A Brief History of Autism

Throughout history there have been accounts of certain behaviors, mannerisms and personal characteristics which we now recognize as being unique to autism/ADHD by both contemporaries and biographers of some famous-and not-so-famous people. A few of these are Microsoft founder, Bill Gates, artist Vincent Van Gogh, filmmakers, Steven Spielberg and Tim Burton, Michelangelo, the great physicists Albert Einstein and Nikola Tesla, mathematician Paul Dirac all of whom-and others- we'll look at again from time to time. Others include Steve Jobs, the English writer, Virginia Woolf along with American actress Daryl Hannah, and Bill Murray,

The word "Autism" itself has its root in the ancient Greek word "autos" meaning of or in "The self." This is the first, vital clue to the understanding of an autistic person. Their situation is such that they are forced by nature to "live inside themselves" to a far greater degree than non-Autists. It is not selfish or by choice; it is a form of isolation and self-containedness, of being imprisoned or "closed off" within oneself. It is no coincidence that the word "automaton"—a robot, comes from the same linguistic root.

There is a very unresponsive, expressionless quality about most Autists which is noticeable as is an absence of physical feedback (Non Verbal Communication-abbreviated by psychologists as NVC-a.k.a "Body Language") particularly in finding the correct interpretations of facial expressions and body posture such as boredom, anger, distress or worry in social settings. These situations are hard or even impossible for Autists to deal with, they cannot break out of themselves no matter how hard they try; however as this book will show, it is often possible, with effort, to break into their world. It is akin to deep-mining for gold and then finding it: an experience which can be deeply rewarding (and in the right circumstances, achingly romantic-the inside of the Special Mind is an intriguing and very different world, compared with normal people) for everyone involved. I'm sure many readers will identify with that experience; Autists are special indeed in many ways.

Autists are people who are definably different from the majority in some well understood and quantifiable ways. The number and types of these ways lie within The Autistic Spectrum, hence Autistic Spectrum Disorders (ASDs). Their symptomatic presentations are many and are rated as 1 "mild," 2 "moderate," 3 "severe" or 4 "profound," according to their degree of influence on the social and physical functionality of the person and the likelihood of their impact on others.

Several of the conditions listed in the spectrum are well known e.g. Dyslexia, derived from the Greek word "dys" meaning "bad," and "lexia," "words." Dyscalculia has the same root, but refers to numbers. Among other presentations on the spectrum are Attention Deficit Disorder, (ADD) Attention Deficit Hyperactive Disorder (ADHD) Asperger's Syndrome, (AS), Pervasive Developmental Disorders-Not Otherwise Specified (PDD-NOS), Williams Syndrome, Hyperlexia, Dyspraxia, High Function Autism, Crohn's Disease and many more. Hyperlexia is an especial fluency and ability with words, written or spoken, a gift many writers, actors and politicians possess, including Winston Churchill and the famous Pulitzer Prize-winning *Washington Post* music critic, Tim Page.

Hyperlexia is found most notably in Asperger's and ADHD people, we'll use the term "Aspies" from now on to describe them. Dyspraxia means being physically uncoordinated – clumsiness and is by no means unique to Autists and pretty normal up to adulthood. Children aren't fully coordinated until they are fully grown.

Moving on to more modern times the words "autism" and "schizophrenia" were both coined around 1911 by a pioneering Swiss psychiatrist named Eugen Bleuler, having noticed "autism" as a particular sub-set of behaviors-now called a "Constellation of symptoms," common to a minority of his group of schizophrenic patients. That was very unfortunate timing as things turned out.

Much against Dr. Bleuler's intentions (he had noted equally "autism" among non-schizophrenics as well) the two conditions became almost inseparably linked in the public mind, due mainly to irresponsible and sensationalist news reporting. This has stigmatized autism by ignorantly demonizing Schizophrenia and has led to a totally unfounded and unreasonable fear of and prejudice against both groups which persists even today both within some sections of the medical and psychiatric community and numerous people in the world outside it. There is a belief that Schizophrenia/Autism = Violent Personality.

The reality is that both groups are far LESS likely to commit either violent or non-violent crimes than "normal" members of society. BUT they are far more likely to be the victims of it. See: https://www.theatlantic.com/health/archive/2012/12/autism-is-not-psychosis/266434/

This is probably due to both the ICD and DSMV correctly listing social dysfunction or periods of social dysfunction as one of their diagnostic criteria for both disorders. We should not therefore discount the strong possibly that autism and schizophrenia, although very different in nature and presentation may be related to each other, that is, they may share some of the same genes or genetic coding, in the same way as Lemon and Lime trees are related, as members the Citrus fruit family.

For many years in psychiatry it was argued that Asperger's is a high-functioning form of schizophrenia. As knowledge increased from the end of the 1950's it became clear that this argument- although understandable at the time- was unsupported and that Asperger's appeared more related to Autism, **and is now recognized in the DSMV as being part of the Autism Spectrum.**

A little earlier these same types of symptoms in non-schizophrenic people had also been identified by a Russian Neurologist, (A

21

specialist in the physical and chemical structures and communication pathways of the brain) Dr. Grunya Sukerava in a book published in 1926, but she did not specifically use the term "Autism" for them. Meanwhile during the same period another Psychiatrist, Emil Kraepelin working at the University of Leipzig in Germany with a mixed group of patients who exhibited many of those same "Constellations" of Symptoms published a book of his observations and theories in 1927 in which he did use the term "autism." The "Constellation" is the unique "signature cluster" of symptoms that identifies any specific condition or Syndrome within the Spectrum as clinically diagnosable.

The next step forward was made in the 1940's by a child psychiatrist working at the Johns Hopkins hospital in Maryland, USA. Dr. Leo Kanner who also used the term autism in two pioneering books to describe his subset of children who exhibited the specific autistic social and emotional traits-which incidentally-he believed were caused by what he termed "Refrigerator Mothers." Meaning, those mothers who could neither nurture nor respond emotionally appropriately to their child's needs. We now know how wrong this was, and it placed a lot of needless guilt on two generations of women throughout the world. Irrespectively, by the end of the 1950's the word "Autism" was widely used in psychiatric practice and its meaning regarding those specific social and emotional problems was generally accepted and understood. International observations had proved that autism was in no way a coincidence and existed independently of other conditions.

At the same time as Dr. Kanner was working in America, an Austrian child specialist, Dr. Hans Asperger was studying yet another group of children at the University of Vienna. He also used the term "autism" and published a major book on the subject in 1944. Concurrently he had noticed both within himself and a very small number of the boys in his care, a variation of autism; a small "Cluster" of symptoms some of which differed greatly from the usual pattern- one, and this is another frequently overlooked trait of Asperger's- is that Aspies naturally speak without a lot of noticeable inflection, in either a sing-song or a monotone voice.

Either can make them seem dull or disinterested, neither of which is true. To these boys he allotted extra time and study. Of that group of four boys, one became a Professor of Astronomy and a second won the Nobel Prize for literature. He died aged 74 in 1980. A year later, a Psychiatrist, Dr. Wing, named that unique sub-cluster after him-coining the highly controversial term "Asperger's Syndrome".

The biggest breakthroughs in the understanding of autism have come from the fields of genetics and brain imaging, notably PET scans, and didn't occur until the late 1980's. They were followed, rapidly by studies in the 90's, until today the heritability of autism and the other Neuro-diverse conditions is an established fact.

This doesn't mean that all forms of autism are always inherited, various other reasons, one being the spontaneous mutation of genes can cause it. Spontaneous mutations happen when an unknown factor or factors cause autistic gene coding to appear in a child whose family has no history of Autism. Some of these probable factors we'll discuss later in the book.

Chapter 2: What is Autism?

Autism should only be diagnosed by a highly qualified specialist with several years of practical and professional experience. Sadly, a number of school and local authority psychiatrists and psychologists who are now giving out record numbers of autism diagnoses have neither. This is one of the reasons behind the much-publicized headline "The Autism Epidemic" and stories of a 6000% rise in cases. This is simply not true-there is no "epidemic" of Autism. There is a rise, but it is not outside the normal variables. In many instances the diagnosis is simply wrong due to the self-styled "expert" being under-qualified or unsuitable to make it; that includes a worryingly large number of completely unqualified people "self-diagnosing" and "diagnosing" their children to get attention, publicity or social/financial benefits. Even when someone has been diagnosed as autistic, it does not mean that they are, as several other conditions can mimic-to the non-expert-the signs of autism. We'll examine some of those conditions in more detail later, but first, we should answer the question "How common is Autism?" It is thought that about five percent of people have a few autistic traits, and about half of those have enough to make them noticeable but not to affect their everyday lives. About 1% only are seen as currently autistic enough to be diagnosed from their symptoms being both numerous and obvious enough to impact their lives and the lives of those around them, according to the Autism Society of America.

There are however Neurodiversity "hot spots" which have grown up over the last three generations, where the number of children born neurodiverse is significantly higher than the average. Why? As we've seen, autism can give a person special skills which are particularly helpful in high tech and mathematics, including programming and robotics. To take one example, since the decision was taken to center the development of the first atom bomb in Palo Alto in San Francisco-the Manhattan Project- that area drew in ultra-clever people from all over the world. After the war the tech continued to develop into space exploration and computing, drawing in even more clever people until it created the tech hub now called "Silicon Valley." That very tight-knit community intermarried and produced another very ND generation, who in turn also intermarried into that same community to the present day. Interestingly, Billionaire founder of PayPal, Peter Thiel had this to say in a 2014 interview with Joe Antenucci...*"One of the strange things in Silicon Valley is that so many of these successful entrepreneurs suffer from a mild form of Asperger's or something like that. And I always think of this as an incredible indictment of our society: What sort of society is it where, if you do not have Asperger's, you will pick up on all these social cues that discourage you from pursuing creative original ideas?"*

Of course, the answer lies in having education systems that impose conformity over creativity-and "Leveling" instead of excelling. That is another reason why most NDs are ignored, persecuted or feared by society, they don't conform—they question and may rebel.

There are other hot spots around the world in Shanghai, China, Seoul in S Korea and Cambridge in England. This again proves that Autism/AS is genetically inherited and that a very few well explained hot spots producing high AS figures do not amount to an Epidemic of Autism outside those tiny areas.

****

Diagnosis:

The principle even semi-reliable method for diagnosing Autism is a process known as "differential diagnosis" (Referred to as "DDx") – the slow investigation and ticking-off of symptoms common to several different possible causes, one-by-one until only the root problem remains.

It is costly and time consuming, while not always right, because it is "diagnosis by exclusion" rather than one by bio-clinical test or scanned imaging. Until very recently it wasn't possible to see or test for autism.

The first time the DDX method was applied in the mental health field was by Dr. Kraepelin.

A proper diagnosis can only be made after an extended study of the patient on the basis of experience and the diagnostic requirements (the Constellation of symptoms) as laid down in the two internationally agreed guides defining what constitute any illness. Plus a degree of instinct by the practitioner, particularly as psychology is not an exact, repeatable science in the way that physics or chemistry are. We should always bear that in mind. There are NO hard and fast scientific tests for any mental illness in the way that there are for purely physical ones such as food poisoning or cholesterol levels, which makes **having the right psychologist or diagnostician even more important-a point that cannot be overstated.**

The two leading international guides referred to are firstly the International Classification of Diseases (ICD) compiled and updated by the World Health Organization (WHO) and covering the diagnostic criteria for all known conditions. Secondly, dealing only with mental conditions is the Diagnostic and Statistical Manual of mental disorders (DSM) published by the American Psychiatric Association (APA). It is by these two books that most psychologists are trained and make their decisions, right or wrong, which is why we need to know them; to understand how the Psychologist is seeing and thinking. That is why parts of them are included in this book, so that adult Autists and parents of autistic children can see what is really going on, along with some explanation of the meanings and consequences of their language. Both agree broadly about autism, with the DSMV defining it as consisting, (slightly abridged), of:

I. A total of six (or more) items from (A), (B), and (C), with at least two from (A), and one each from (B) and (C)

(A) Qualitative impairment in social interaction, as manifested by at least two of the following:

1. Marked impairments in the use of multiple non-verbal behaviors such as eye-to-eye gaze, facial expression, body posture, and gestures to regulate social interaction.

2. Failure to develop peer relationships appropriate to developmental level:

3. A lack of spontaneous seeking to share enjoyment, interests, or achievements with other people, (e.g., by a lack of showing, bringing, or pointing out objects of interest to other people).

4. lack of social or emotional reciprocity (note: in the description, it gives the following as examples: not actively participating in simple social play or games, preferring solitary activities, or involving others in activities only as tools or "mechanical" aids.)

(B) Qualitative impairments in communication as manifested by at least one of the following:

1. Delay in; or total lack of, the development of spoken language (not accompanied by an attempt to compensate through alternative modes of communication such as gesture or mime).

2. In individuals with adequate speech, a marked inability to sustain a conversation with others.

3 Stereotyped and repetitive use of language or idiosyncratic language.

4. Lack of varied, spontaneous make-believe play or social imitative play appropriate to developmental level.

(C) Restricted repetitive and stereotyped patterns of behavior, interests and activities, as manifested by at least two of the following:

1. An encompassing preoccupation with one or more stereotyped and restricted patterns of interest that is abnormal either in intensity or focus.

2. Apparently inflexible adherence to specific non-functional routines or rituals (OCD-ICH).

3. Stereotyped and repetitive motor mannerisms (e.g. hand or finger flapping or twisting, or complex whole-body movements ("stimming").

4. Persistent preoccupation with parts of objects (for instance mechanical objects).

II. Delays or abnormal functioning in at least one of the following areas, with an onset prior to age 3 years:

1. Social interaction

2. Language as used in social communication

3. Symbolic or imaginative play

III. The disturbance is not better accounted for by Rett's Disorder or Childhood Disintegrative Disorder (CDD).

Before autism can be diagnosed at least two symptoms from A to C must be present permanently and at least one from section III.

Author's Note: Rett's Disorder is a physical disease of and damage to part of the white matter in the brain. It is very rare, always genetic in origin and occurs almost exclusively in girls. The patients have noticeable physical differences from normal children, including very small heads and feet. It is very serious, life-limiting and causes extreme retardation* in most cases-the child can never talk or live any kind of normal or independent life. It is virtually unrelated to autism, although profound autism can closely resemble it in its lack of mental development.

Childhood Disintegrative Disorder (CDD), better known as Heller's Syndrome after Theodore Heller who first described it in 1908. In it the child affected develops normally or even super-normally until somewhere between two and ten years of age and then rapidly regresses to severe dependence from which there is no recovery. It is "Idiopathic," meaning there is no known cause. Like Rett's it can, at certain points in the regression the process resembles autism, although it is not. Worryingly that has not stopped a lot of children with CDD being given the wrong diagnosis and the wrong treatment and that applies equally to Rett's sufferers and their carers.

Retardation:

*The continued use of this long-outdated term by the Psychiatric, Psychological and Medical Establishments is highly inappropriate and deeply offensive for the whole of the Neuro-Diverse **(ND)** community. It does though shed the true, dark light in which these professions still see and treat Neuro-diverse people, whatever their public smiles and honeyed words-it is a warning to us all. My preferred term is "Developmental variances." This situation can only be improved by a thorough overhaul of recruitment practices; better training and understanding within these professions.

The big problem for many children with autism and other developmental variances is that they stop progressing mentally at a certain age. If that is very young, they will remain babies in terms of mental, if not physical capability all their lives and can never communicate nor take care of themselves. They cannot for example, eat, dress or use a bathroom independently. The heartbreak for the parents of such children is agonizing beyond any power of description and they need every possible support; physical, financial and emotional-as do any other "normal" siblings in the family structure. Autism is neither a curse nor a judgment; it's a genetic lottery.

The ICD (Section 10) criteria for an autism diagnosis (slightly abridged) are:

Abnormal or impaired development is evident before the age of 3 years in at least one of the following areas:

(A) Receptive or expressive language as used in social communication.

(B) The development of selective social attachments or of reciprocal social interaction, such as functional or symbolic play.

(C) A total of at least six symptoms from (1), (2) and (3) must be present, with at least two from (1) and at least one from each of (2) and (3) for a diagnosis.

Qualitative impairment in social interaction is manifested in at least two of the following areas:

(A) Failure adequately to use eye-to-eye gaze, facial expression, body postures, and gestures to regulate "normal" social interaction.

(B) Failure to develop (in a manner appropriate to mental age, and despite ample opportunities) peer group (their age) relationships that involve a mutual sharing of interests, activities and emotions.

(C) Lack of socio-emotional reciprocity is shown by an impaired or deviant response to other people's emotions; or lack of modulation of behaviors according to social context; or a weak integration of social, emotional, and communicative behaviors; lack of spontaneous seeking to share enjoyment, interests, or achievements with other people (e.g. a lack of showing, bringing, or pointing out to other people objects of interest to the individual).

Qualitative abnormalities in communication as manifest in at least one of the following areas:

(A) Delay in or total lack of development of spoken language that is not accompanied by an attempt to compensate through the use of gestures or mime as an alternative mode of communication (often preceded by a lack of communicative babbling); *Author's note*: "Baby Talk."

(B) Relative failure to initiate or sustain conversational interchange (at whatever level of language skill is present) in which there is reciprocal responsiveness to the communications of the other person: Stereotyped and repetitive use of language or idiosyncratic use of words or phrases; lack of varied spontaneous make-believe play or (when young) social imitative play

(C) Restricted, repetitive, and stereotyped patterns of behavior, interests, and activities are manifested in at least one of the following;

(D) An encompassing preoccupation with one or more stereotyped and restricted patterns of interest that are abnormal in content or focus; or one or more interests that are abnormal in their intensity and circumscribed nature though not in their content or focus;

(E) Apparently compulsive adherence to specific, nonfunctional routines or rituals.

Author's note: Stacking blocks or other specific object arrangement, such as clothes in a particular drawer, box or order, which if disturbed causes the person of any age great and prolonged distress are examples of such rituals.

****

Stereotyped and repetitive motor mannerisms that involve either hand or finger flapping or twisting or complex whole-body movements…

Author's Note-these movements (Body movements are called "Motor function" by doctors) are known as "stimming" and are usually compulsive, life-long and often done unconsciously and/or involuntarily. It is my belief from years of research and observation that Tourette's Syndrome is part of the autistic family as a verbal form of stimming and that both, along with Obsessive-Compulsive behaviors are greatly magnified by the high levels of well-justified and grounded anxiety (anxiety makes anything worse) which is in almost all cases clearly a product of that person's life situation. In the same way, stammering and facial tics are usually the result of stress-much of it is the fault of the poor or no-care and concern that Autists generally receive from society and not so much because of autism itself or any other psychological disorder. Stimming is usually harmless, and many Autists find it a good way to deal with anxiety, so it should be seen as a positive behavior.

Intense preoccupations with part-objects of non-functional elements of play materials (such as their order of color, their texture, or the vibration/movement they generate).

The clinical picture is not attributable to the other varieties of pervasive developmental disorders; specific development disorder of receptive language with secondary socio-emotional problems, reactive attachment disorder or dis-inhibited attachment disorder.

Author's note: this means the child's current physical and/or emotional environment.

Mental retardation with some associated emotional or behavioral disorders; schizophrenia of unusually early onset; and Rett's Syndrome:

****

As can be seen, they are both very similar in emphasis and give together a reasonably complete picture of autistic behavior and traits-namely of someone "living in their head" and taking little if any interest in the people or world outside themselves to a noticeable extent-even to the point where-and this has to be said-the person, whether an adult or child is so "Frozen" and withdrawn that they need lifelong institutional care—it depends on the type and severity of the autism. It also illustrates the process of DDx.

Autistic Fact: As both children and adults, Autists frequently reject both contact and gifts from family and friends, which can cause feelings of failure, hurt and alienation, particularly to parents. **This behavior is not a rejection.** Autists by-and-large don't like being touched and may refuse cuddles and hugs-because they are very sensitive to them- it may be constricting or even painful. Autistics have very different pain thresholds from NTs, something that doctors and care workers need to realize. With regard to presents-essentially expressions of love- they will either totally get into the Autist's world or not at all. It's not personal, they do love you, so don't be saddened by it, it's just a fact of the condition. Conversely if a toy, even a cheap simple trinket or piece of material really "locks" the Autist's interest, it can become a lifelong talisman and companion- & very satisfying for the giver. Some you win, some you lose. :) None of this means that a person's quality of life cannot be improved by the strategies we'll come to examine later, regardless of the setting in which they are practiced.

Yet things are not quite so cut and dried as was thought when those manuals were first written and approved, more than two decades ago. Researchers in the fields of biomedicine, biophysics and genetics have opened up exciting new questions and answers which have necessitated both a substantial re-thinking and updating of our ideas of Neuro-diversity in general and add surely another further imperative to finding the right diagnosis and the best therapies.

Chapter 3: What is Asperger's Syndrome?

Asperger's Syndrome (AS) is still, in many parts of the world considered independently as a branch of Autism sharing many of its characteristics with other identifiable conditions like Schizophrenia but also with its own unique indications, making it a separate condition, as shown in the "illustrations section." The DSM (V) lists the criteria within the Autism section, as...

I. Qualitative impairment in social interaction, as manifested by at least two of the following:

(A) Marked impairments in the use of multiple non-verbal behaviors such as eye-to-eye gaze, facial expression, body posture, and gestures to regulate social interaction.

(B) Failure to develop peer relationships appropriate to developmental level

(C) A lack of spontaneous seeking to share enjoyment, interest or achievements with other people, (e.g. by a lack of showing, bringing, or pointing out objects of interest to other people)

(D) Lack of social or emotional reciprocity (*Author's note*: social give-and-take)

II. Restricted repetitive & stereotyped patterns of behavior, interests and activities, as manifested by at least one of the following:

(A) Encompassing preoccupation with one or more stereotyped and restricted patterns of interest that is abnormal either in intensity or focus.

(B) Apparently inflexible adherence to specific, nonfunctional routines or rituals.

(C) Stereotyped and repetitive motor mannerisms (e.g. hand or finger-flapping or twisting) Again, complex whole-body movements.

(D) Persistent preoccupation with parts of objects (Like watch mechanisms-author).

III. The disturbance causes clinically significant impairments in social, occupational, or other important areas of functioning.

IV. There is no clinically significant general delay in language e.g. single words used by age 2 years, communicative phrases used by age 3 Years) there is no clinically significant delay in cognitive development or in the development of age-appropriate self-help skills, adaptive behavior (other than in social interaction) and curiosity about the environment in childhood.

Author's Note: "Cognitive" just means the ability to think and understand here.

Criteria are not met for another specific Pervasive Developmental Disorder or Schizophrenia.

****

And by the ICD as:

(A) Lack of any clinically significant general delay in spoken or receptive language or cognitive development: Diagnosis requires that single words should have developed by two years of age or earlier and that communicative phrases are used by three years of age or earlier. Self-help skills, adaptive behavior and curiosity about the environment during the first three years should be at a level consistent with intellectual development. However, motor milestones may be somewhat delayed and motor clumsiness is usual (although not a necessary diagnostic feature). Isolated special skills, often related to abnormal preoccupations, are common, but are not required for diagnosis. I didn't speak at all until nearly 48 months, quite significantly late, the usual being 12-18 months, but as my Mum said, "once you did, we couldn't stop you." :)

(B) Qualitative abnormalities in reciprocal social interaction (criteria as for autism).

(C) An unusually intense circumscribed interest or restrictive, repetitive, and stereotyped patterns of behavior, interests and activities (criteria as for autism; however, it would be less usual for these to include either motor mannerisms or preoccupations with part-objects or non-functional elements of play materials). (*Author's note*, I used to love taking mechanical toys, clocks, locks and small electric motors apart as a kid).

(D) The disorder is not attributable to other varieties of pervasive developmental disorder; schizoid-type disorder, simple schizophrenia; reactive and dis-inhibited attachment disorder of childhood (F94.1 and 2).

Obsessional personality disorder (OPD) or obsessive-compulsive disorder (OCD).

Author's note: "Attributable" is a matter of personal opinion; it's a "maybe," not hard science and therefore too subjective to be generally reliable. It's always worth seeking more than one opinion as these may vary considerably in quality and helpfulness, as well as accuracy.

These two guides, however, along with other professional manuals and from the professional communities around the world remain very much in baseline agreement.

However, there is one *caveat*; the DSM IV is still widely used today although it was replaced by version five in May 2013. It removes Asperger's Syndrome as a separate category while putting its entire and unique profile list within the Autism section. That is viewed by some, especially in Europe and Asia with deep suspicion for the fact that it is composed of only ONE specialized profession. It is not multidisciplinary as the ICD is and therefore not as comprehensive or independently checked for errors. By others it is still held in high regard. The ICD, which does recognize Asperger's as a separate condition, is now in its tenth version, having always been updated more frequently than the DSMs and being an independently globally resourced work has always been my diagnostic manual of choice.

Case Study 1: We have noticed that one of the many factors uniting Autism and AS is the concentration on, and love of, repetitive behavior-which doesn't have to be a bad thing- as this case illustrates. An ADD client of mine works in the critical field of large-structure shot-blasting and protective painting in harsh environments. It is highly skilled and highly detailed work.

For example, the humidity has to be EXACTLY right and needs very sensitive electronic measurement or the protective paint won't stick. It is also very repetitive, repainting the same structures is an unending (if well paid) task, which demands immense and purposeful concentration, as one tiny "miss," a micron or two of paint too thin could lead directly to the entire assembly being fatally weakened and hundreds or perhaps thousands of people killed. He enjoys exactly that kind of environment with no "hands-on" supervision, no set hours and total attention to detail with precise repetition. For him being an Autist makes him perfect for that job and us a lot safer. Personally, he is a really good bloke who prefers having friends round, more than going out to social meeting places.

What is so special about Asperger s?

The answer to that now commonly asked question is very complex, to begin with we must look both outside and behind the dry academic covers of the DSMs and ICD to reveal the first, hidden secrets of Autism and AS.

Firstly, it must be remembered that overt autism is very uncommon, only that previously mentioned 1-ish%.

One of the few aspects of autism that is appealing is that statistic. It remains constant throughout every country, racial, cultural and social grouping so far examined. That fact alone of autism existing is one of the defining proofs of our shared humanity and hopefully banishes once and for all any thoughts or acts of racial bias or so-called "social superiority," which are still seen and heard all too often even today. Unfortunately, these attitudes do exist and result in even more people of minority communities being ignored or marginalized and going undiagnosed and untreated-this needs to stop. Those of us—who are able to—should stand up and draw attention to this situation and demand an end to all inequality. Autism is both part of and proof of our shared humanity and heritage.

The number of true, full-blown Aspies is a subject of open debate and on-going study, so a single defining figure is not yet possible. My research over more than 20 years suggests a figure of around one in seventeen or eighteen thousand Autists only, it's very, very rare, one in 18,000 of only 2% (at most) of the population. Aspies have certain differences from other autistics, as well as much in common with them.

Firstly, because an Aspie is in most cases physically and developmentally normal-although they quite often learn to speak and co-ordinate a little later than the average child, boy or girl - they are not otherwise obviously abnormal-except, as the books say, they do not have the standard social skills (or sometimes any) and responses, or understanding of them. They live outside the mainstream social box. Asperger's Syndrome is to the greatest degree a SOCIAL disorder, without intellectual impairment-and that is our first great secret, additionally, an Aspie may occasionally have some very special talent.

Another myth surrounding autism that needs to be dispelled is that Autists are anti-or asocial. One of the things which makes autism/AS so hard for a person- I never use the term "sufferer" in referring to Autism/AS because they are not diseases or illnesses-is the communication difficulty with social life.

It's hard to make friends and form other deep relationships, even with parents and close family members due to that "closed inness."

That secretiveness and reclusiveness alienates the world. Autists are often seen as sly, shy, arrogant, aloof, or simply detached and uncaring and as a result are denied the opportunities to become part of an organization, group or whatever. They are adrift, often painfully alone and unable to use whatever talents they possess to benefit and contribute to society-a thing which almost all I have met desperately want to do—to fit in and to help (we are not lazy) to love and to be loved. **We want to be seen, accepted and recognized for who we are, not side-lined for what we are not.**

There are, unfortunately a few able Autists who feel, "I'm autistic, I have nothing to offer." Nonsense! Everyone has something to offer, and I urge everyone to try. There is nothing wrong with failure, but there is in not trying. By trying we often learn much about ourselves and achieve far more than we ever thought possible. We can all do something, no matter how large or small (That's not important). That it is a far richer and more satisfying life than sitting back and doing nothing, is the important thing.

In the matter of close interpersonal relationships, Autists can't recognize another person's interest in them-they need to be told directly-and find it hard to "reach out" appropriately, socially, sexually and intellectually. As a result, we are frequently mistrusted and friendless, almost "invisible", denied that of which the Roman Statesman, Lawyer and Philosopher Cicero wrote of friendship two thousand years ago:

"What is sweeter than to have someone with whom you may dare discuss anything, as if communing with your own self...Adversity would indeed be hard to bear without him to whom the burden would be heavier than to oneself."

Having an autistic child makes life hard on the family, who also get pushed away and ignored by mainstream society, which cannot, (or will not) handle autism. For this reason, I cannot speak too highly or warmly of many of the largely voluntary self-help and support groups that have grown up over the last twenty years. Autism is a heavy and often solitary struggle at any age.

Aspie-spotting: Aspies can often be spotted by the way they dress-we like loose-fitting, soft clothing, brushed cotton for example and tend to go for high neck clothes for both men and women, with a preference for light, monochrome pastel colors.

Aspies are different. Across a large sample of any randomly chosen group, people with AS are, on average, 10% more intelligent than their peers. The average person has an IQ of 100, the average Aspie has an IQ of about 110-the same applies across the whole range of intelligence-also their Verbal IQ -the ability to put thoughts into words-is higher again. This does not mean of course that all Aspies are geniuses, some profoundly affected ones have very low IQ's-perhaps only 70, which is a severe disability, but across the board they are smarter and talk/write better than the average-which can cause a jealousy reaction, often leading to bullying in schools and workplaces.

It is for this reason that Aspie children are often teased as "little professors," a term originally used of them by Dr. Asperger himself (and of myself by classmates and teachers, since about the age of 6) which is very isolating giving me an "I don't fit in," feeling that has left its psychological scars. Most autistic people have been emotionally damaged in some way or another. It is related to their extraordinary capacity to absorb, memorize/process and relay information about the topics which interest them, coupled with the extreme ability to "shut the world out" and focus deeply into those topics.

Several highly respected authorities have stated that there are advantages to the individual in being autistic at certain Function Levels, especially in being Asperger's which is widely regarded as the "mildest" form on the Autistic Spectrum Disorders.

The most notable among these is perhaps the 2002 Nobel prize-winning economist, Dr. Vernon Smith, currently Professor of Economics and Law at Chapman University California. Rather than putting it as an appendix or summarizing, it is worth quoting at some length an interview given by Dr. Smith to CBNC, an American Television Channel in 2003. It helps contextualize part of the motivation for this work: namely, an attempt to delve more deeply into both the socioeconomics and the many ambiguities underpinning Autism—the gap between the autistic's self-perception and the perception of them held by others.

****

Preamble: "People with Asperger's often have extreme difficulty interacting socially, preferring to focus on narrow fields of interest. But often they're able to pursue those interests with great intensity…" – CBNC

Smith: "I can switch out and go into a concentrated mode and the world is completely shut out…If I'm writing something, nothing else exists… Perhaps even more importantly, I don't have any trouble thinking outside the box. I don't feel any social pressure to do things the way other people are doing them, professionally. And so I have been more open to different ways of looking at a lot of the problems in economics."

CBNC: Did you feel like you seemed strange in the eyes of other people?

Smith: Oh, yes.

CBNC: How so?

Smith: Sometimes I'm described as being "not there" in a social situation. You know a social situation that lasts for a couple of hours I find it to be a tremendous amount of strain, so I've been known just to go to bed and read.

Dr. Smith's wife has described him as follows: "I could not understand why he cannot be any part of my emotional world. He might not always know what he feels...In fact, many times he doesn't. He'll say, "I don't know. What do you mean? ...Many people don't understand Vernon and they conclude wrongly about him."

This conversational evidence illuminates a crucial point about a major diagnostic criterion; that Asperger's really is primarily a cognitive, social disorder as Dr. Brosnan *et al* of Bath University in the UK stated in the *Journal of Child Psychology and Psychiatry* in 2004.

Maybe that is not such an issue for a wealthy, prize-winning economist; however, in my experience Asperger's and autism have more downsides than up. Two points in particular that arise from the interview are worth noting. It illustrates the gulf between Dr. Smith's self-image–that even though he's different, it is, by his own implication all to the good- and that which others have of him, i.e. that he is "Strange." Indeed, AS is often referred to in street slang as *"Strange man syndrome."* Aspies are certainly individualists who best march to the beat of their own drum and are always the happiest and most successful when accorded the freedom to do so.

Secondly, Mrs. Smith's highly astute comment concerning people drawing the wrong conclusions about her husband sums up the experience of most Aspies well, as does that frequently echoed word "strange." We are often misunderstood (Myself included). It is in part this "strangeness" that can and often does lead to the ignoring, abuse and persecution of autistic people and their families by mainstream society. To guard against the ignorant, all Autists should learn a martial art, not only for fitness and self-defense but for the extra self-confidence, philosophy and self-discipline which are learned along with them. Tae-Kwon-Do was my choice at age 18, I wish it had been earlier.

(CBNC) Some doctors who treat people with Asperger's like Dr. Ami Klin at Yale University... (Have a different perspective) "Dr. Smith's success is not typical of most people with this disability. The vast majority of individuals with Asperger Syndrome need help-without that help they won't be able to do very well... "The individuals that I know have to overcome a great deal of difficulty to maximize their potential and get the things in life they deserve," says Dr. Klin. Most of that difficulty is caused by the lack of meaningful social understanding between Aspies and NTs. Aspies aren't good at expressing things-including their feelings and needs, in clinical terms that inability is called Alexythemia.

Dr. Smith is, of course right, proven not only by his own remarkable story, but by those of other notable Aspie and Autistic high achievers. Furthermore, an important and wide-ranging research project headed by Dr. Larry Cahill in 2006 from the University of California in Irvine, showed that people who have unusually large development in certain sectors of the brain, particularly near the Left temporoparietal junction region have exceptional memory capacity and recall. Interestingly that same development is also associated with OCD (Obsessional Compulsive Disorder), an acknowledged member of the Autism Spectrum which is also common.

That said, the day-to-day life experience of most autistic/AS and other Neuro-diverse people agrees far more closely with Dr. Klin's view than with Dr. Smith's. Being an Aspie is generally not great fun, mainly due to the interpersonal relationship issues and discrimination already discussed which tends to go along with it, as well as the lack of help and empathy from mainstream society. Because we look pretty "normal" and tend to "mask" our Condition and feelings-that is- try to copy and act "normal," to try to "fit in", only a few people see us as needing help. But we do need it in many areas all the time as Dr. Klin explained. "Masking" is a form of acting, of that ability to imitate, pretending to be OK, when we're not, but don't know how to "reach out" for help, so it's very dangerous in some circumstances. It also takes a huge amount of mental, physical and emotional energy which can suck you dry and burnt out.

The question of whether the reason for that is clinical or social is not yet answered, but the majority of my clients and friends feel that if autism/AS had been a seasonal gift, like a birthday or Christmas present, they would have hoped it came with the receipt; so that they could exchange it for something...perhaps a little more fun and comfortable?

At this point let's pause and take a look at another false assumption made by certain sections of the mass media and medical/education professionals; namely that so-called HFA (High Functioning Autism) and Asperger's Syndrome are the same thing, they're not! It is not true that all HFAs are Aspies nor that all Aspies are HFAs. A radical modern re-definition of HFA is urgently needed. I'm gonna do that right now!

"HFA is now the only recognized term to apply to a child or adult who has previously been diagnosed with an Autism Spectrum Disorder and additionally exhibits a Performance IQ of over 130." (I. Hale).

With reference to Performance IQ: The following scale is widely used. 110-130 = "bright" 130-150 = "gifted" 150-170 = "genius" 170 + = "hyper-genius," 200+ "Super-genius."

The use of the term "Performance IQ" is with reference to Professor Howard Gardner's (From Harvard University, USA) *Theory of Multiple Intelligences* (1983), a brilliant and ground-breaking work on intelligence, child potential and education. Basically, some people are better at some things than others and to different levels of ability in each area. We need this definition otherwise there is an assumption that all Asperger's people are intellectually "gifted," which is not often the case. These children especially can be saddled with an unbearable and unrealistic level of expectation. Every school and parent want an Einstein but that just isn't going to happen.

45

A few Aspies do have special abilities, occasionally far beyond the normal, yet those abilities are often not traditionally academic ones. It does a child a great and permanent disservice to assume ability where none exists and to expect a performance level of which the child may simply not be capable. This can lead to low self-esteem, demotivation, adult depression, and suicide.

It is a grim fact, but one that must not be avoided or made taboo as it has been. Let's break that taboo now and talk about the facts of suicide. Autists in general: are (26 times) and Aspies in particular, (46 times) more likely to commit suicide than the average member of the public; male or female. As a result, the average life expectancy of someone with Autism/AS is only 39 years... the same fact applies to other Neuro-diverse groups. Let that chilling statistic sink in.

Einstein and Edison:

Einstein had super-high intellectual (IQ) function, which is solely how I am defining being HFA-by IQ. But he had the same social and communication problems, including being profoundly dyslexic as any other autistic person. He needed (as all gifted children need) specialist help at school to fulfil his genius-which, like so many, then and now, he didn't get. From the age of 12 he became largely self-taught. Einstein remained bitter over his wasted, wretched school years all his life, which influenced his later, playful, engaging and energetic style of teaching-in stark contrast to the regimented, narrow schooling he had received.

Another equally famous example is Thomas Edison, another brilliant autistic who was unappreciated and finally expelled from the school system. Fortunately, his Mother was a strong, amazing and clever woman who home-schooled young Thomas to fulfil his full potential. Homeschooling is, again today becoming an increasingly popular option exercised by families because of the failure of mainstream education to protect and nurture their child's talents or needs, the "deep mining for gold" we agreed on earlier.

Rigid, mainstream, state education doesn't work for special children. I totally support homeschooling by qualified parents or a certified locum community teacher.

Bearing this in mind, we should be aware that even the most up to date of modern IQ tests are still short of being a perfectly honed and proven scientific tool. We would be wise not to place all our faith in them, despite their constant development and improvement giving us an increasingly accurate picture. This is especially true when they are used in combination with Psychometric personality testing, which assesses various strengths and weaknesses and is very accurate these days, aided by Psychiatric assessment. Still, **the truth is we still can't define what "Intelligence" actually is in concrete terms.** It is always, at least in part, a slippery social and cultural construct. What is now well understood is that there is a strong inherited component to IQ, as explained in the work of Professor Paul Thompson of the University of California in Los Angeles (UCLA) published in 2012. There are inherently "smart families," as there are inherently "Autistic/AS families," quite often they are one in the same.

Regardless of that, it is also vitally important to keep in mind a moral perspective as well as the intellectual one. Because a person has a low IQ by today's criteria does not in the least diminish their value as a human being. Nor does it necessarily mean their lives will be empty, unhappy or unproductive unless society makes them so.

That comment applies equally to those at the opposite end of the IQ scale, whom society tends to mistrust or fear because they are too "different," or "too clever by half," leaving them without the physical and emotional support they so badly need, as Dr. Klin noted. People are frightened by what they don't understand.

Those geniuses whether autistic or NT are very rare, but when they do occur, the Aspie/ Autist type, like Dr. Smith and others seem to have, by precedent that little extra spark of insightfulness and original thinking born of the ability to focus so intently on whatever they are doing and thinking without socially constructed preconceptions-outside the box. It seems to give them an edge over the rest, perhaps that edge is what society calls "creativity"? None of this is intended to imply that HFAs are the only members of the Autistic Family who can excel in some way.

There are many very "Gifted Autistics" who are not HFA and whose gifts reside beyond the purely intellectual, like mathematics, literature or economics. Theirs perhaps are in sculpture, STEM crafts, sports or painting—these being six well-recognized areas in which some Autists, whether Aspies or not, have done exceptionally well. There are of course geniuses in every field who are not in the slightest bit autistic: but to paraphrase a well-known Autism Community joke: "you don't have to be an autist to be a genius, but it does help." :)

Aspie Fact: myth-Aspies don't have a sense of humor. Most of us do, if only as a defense mechanism and a medium of stress relief. A few NTs find Aspie humor too clever, ironic, dark or inappropriate in certain situations, which can cause problems, as can the fact that we don't laugh or smile much and sometimes find it hard to understand and appreciate sarcasm and especially jokes centering on words or phrases having double-meanings, or specific physical gestures. The message to people who think we lack humor is "take a good look at yourself first!"

****

No doubt some readers will disagree about Dyslexia having been included without a *caveat* earlier, in the Autistic Spectrum, when it is often classed as a Non-Verbal Learning Disability (NLD). It does though frequently present with Autism, although it may not always be autistic in origin. The reason behind this inclusion is that I have never met anyone with Asperger's or HFA who does not present at the same time, at least some degree of Dyslexia as well. Nor have I found any one of those two with just a single tell-tale Autistic characteristic. Usually there is the main defining one, with at least two additional sub-characteristics of varying severity. For example: Asperger's plus some degree of ADHD and/or Dyslexia and so on. In most professionals' opinion, Dyslexia can be either purely autistic or NLD in origin.

Note: Non-verbal in NLD means that the person's speech is normal, but there are other problems, like reading difficulty. In another context, it means not being able to speak at all.

Everyone involved in educational assessment should guard against an over-hasty Dyslexia-only diagnosis and should look for Autistic characteristics as well as possible visual or hearing impairments as the underlying cause. It is all too easy to be presented with apparent Dyslexia and look no further.

It should be a matter of the gravest concern that so many Autists have passed through education systems un-noticed due to an uninformed or incomplete diagnosis of Dyslexia as an NLD. Sometimes the two are hard to tell apart, but that does not make failing to do so any more professionally acceptable. Throughout my career I have interviewed students who came with Dyslexia "Statements," only to notice that ADHD or ADD were also present, making them much more likely to be Autistic than NLD. That omission will usually have a deeply negative effect on their educational provision, experience and standard.

Conversely, we must also recognize that in certain countries schools get extra money for every extra "dyslexic/dyspraxic/autistic" pupil enrolled. That leads to an unhealthy and unprofessional relationship between the school, the Board of Governors, the funding agency and the education psychologist. I have witnessed this corruption in operation and seen children falsely "labelled" for life. It makes me angry.

Bluntly, I have seen schools and colleges pay psychologists to diagnose normal children for extra funding which ends up in the Head teacher's and governor's pockets.

****

Now let us again correct another damaging myth about Neurodiversity: namely that people with Asperger's Syndrome/Schizophrenia are more dangerous than the average member of the public and are more likely to commit violent crime. Totally false:

That is the conclusion of a major project, *dispelling the Stigma of Schizophrenia*: By David L. Penn, Samatha Kommana, Maureen Mansfield, and Bruce Q. Link, published in the *Schizophrenia Bulletin*, Vol. 25, No. 3, 1999. "People often fear individuals with schizophrenia because they believe that the disorder is linked to violent behavior." However, the research concluded that there is only a weak association between **any** major psychiatric/ND disorder and violence in the community.

Furthermore, recent studies suggest that individuals who abuse drugs or alcohol are hugely more likely to be violent than individuals with schizophrenia. Specifically, the prevalence of violence is highest among individuals who abuse drugs (34.7%).

Numerous other projects before and since back up this team's findings, not only regarding schizophrenics, but the Autism Spectrum as well. Dr. J W Swanson's (of Oxford University) 2006 study came to a similar conclusion. Virtually every study conducted has found that murder rates and other violent crimes are **significantly lower among autistic/AS people than average** and that the same is true of schizophrenics.

The violence delusion originated from and was then twisted by elements in the mass media for the sole purpose of sensationalist, profit-boosting headlines. They deliberately concentrated on the very few violent crimes committed by these groups, without ever contextualizing them by giving comparative figures from other sections of the population. Secondly, they omitted to acknowledge that most violence committed by our three groups is *self-harm*, despite the fact that Schizophrenics, like Aspies are also as, if not more intelligent and insightful than an average person. I feel confident that many people, including families, Autists, doctors, carers and teachers all agree with the view that large sections of the media should be thoroughly ashamed of themselves and their behavior over the years, which has caused so much misery and danger from vigilantism against these already stigmatized and vulnerable groups.

Society should fear the violent crime of drug users; and that particularly relates to alcohol abuse. For example, a leaked (and later verified) UK Government report commissioned by MP Chris Grayling was published in *The Daily Mail,* on April 6, 2010, in an article written by the noted journalist James Black; and the figures are horrifying:

47% of all violent crimes are committed under the influence of alcohol, including domestic violence.

62% of all random unprovoked violence committed on people by total strangers was alcohol-fueled.

36% of all jail entries were caused by alcohol-related offenses including drink-driving.

Alcohol is without any question the primary "gateway drug," that is, the one which leads people on to harder illegal drugs, like solvents, Meth, crack Cocaine, PCP ("Angel Dust"), Ketamine or the opiates, all far worse than cannabis, psilocybin or LSD have ever been. Psilocybin is the active chemical in magic mushrooms and is showing signs of being a very promising treatment for numerous conditions, including healing brain injuries, PTSD, and depression.

That was also the conclusion of several other large-scale surveys. Firstly in 1985 by John Welte and Grace Barnes for New York State University in Buffalo, secondly from Missouri Western State University in 2009, and finally by the world-renowned Prof. David Nutt of Imperial College, London in 2010. He concluded his co-written article in the British medical journal, *The Lancet* (Founded in 1823) by saying... "Overall, alcohol was the most harmful drug (overall harm score 72), with heroin (55) and crack cocaine (54) in second and third places." The main point is that the majority of people use alcohol before using any of the others, which is what makes it and not cannabis the biggest problem as the "gateway drug," aside from all the other negatives we have seen. That said, heavy cannabis use (more than 3 times a week) has been repeatedly shown to reduce IQ and increase the chances of developing mental illness, especially when the users begin young; that is, before their teens or early twenties. The risk among older users is considerably less. Smoking cannabis badly damages your lungs, memory and increases the chances of dementia in later life. There is the possibility that it could equally affect the brains of developing babies whose mothers use the drug during pregnancy, perhaps leading to autism or Learning Difficulties. That is so far unproven, however the message is strongly, "don't take that chance, and don't do street drugs, especially while pregnant and/or breastfeeding" (I. Hale).

To balance that view: There is both a substantial body of scientific and user-experience evidence that *Medical* cannabis extracts, like CBD oils may have a broad range of positive psychological and physical benefits with fewer adverse side effects than many current pharmaceutical drugs.

Some of these benefits may apply to the fields of Autism, anxiety, pain relief and epilepsy and help with sleep. More research is required before coming to a definitive conclusion.

Society should take a long, hard look at its real and not imaginary threats: Primarily alcohol, but also the highly stimulant behavior-altering drugs that include Cocaine and Methamphetamines as the causes of serious crime and stop the witch-hunt against those who are already themselves, innocent victims of certain, mainly harmless, if obvious mental conditions. A prime message of this book is, "please look at the facts first-not the trash end of the media- before making judgments about Autism in particular or mental health in general."

As an Aspie friend put it rightly when she said, "I don't have a problem with being Asperger's. It's other people who have a problem with me being Asperger's."

Chapter 4: The Significance of Autism/Asperger's Syndrome

We need to begin this chapter with a re-cap of how Autism is diagnosed: Briefly if anyone at any age exhibits a sufficient number of the criteria unique to autism, as defined by the ICD or the DSM then the correct diagnosis is "autism" once other potential causes have been ruled out. The patient can then, according to which and to how big an extent he/she has their symptoms, be told exactly which autistic condition or conditions they have and where they are in the Autistic Family and therefore find the most appropriate help. At least that's how the system is supposed to work.

But...Autism has two faces, dependent (usually) on its likely cause and defined largely by the age at which it first presents-that is-becomes noticeable to the parents and a doctor- to a point where it's clear that the child is "different." In practice, someone especially close to the child, usually the mother instinctively knows if her baby is different much earlier than the three years cited in the manuals. My Mum noticed before I was two.

There is only "Classical Autism," the cause of which is wholly genetic and is always apparent before the age of three, as both the DSM and ICD agree.

The other autism-like conditions like NLDs; are best explained in Sue Thompson's excellent (1996) book *The Source for Non-Verbal Learning Disorders* (NLDs). Not only is it an invaluable practical manual (and highly recommended from my experience for all SEN teachers and carers alike) but it also explains precisely both the nature of NLDs and the underlying science behind the conditions which separates them from the genetically induced childhood autism. She explains in the book, how some children (and adults) develop autism symptoms across the whole age range for very specific reasons that we'll examine in the next chapter.

These cases are referred to as Non-Verbal Learning Disorders to distinguish them from inherited "classical" autism or acquired "non-classical" autism. Sometimes the two are impossible to tell apart, except (and then not always) by genetic testing, blood analysis (usually for heavy metals) and PER brain-scanning, because although the causes are different, the observable effects are often very similar.

To complicate things a little further: (That sentence itself would serve as an appropriate motto for dealing with autism), children without autistic genes can be exposed to the other causes of autism before the age of three. Without genetic testing such children may be classified as having classical autism, which is medically incurable, despite the many fake claims to the contrary which are continually made. The people who make these claims are dangerous, greedy liars and some of their so-called "cures" like MMS ("bleaching") and electric shocking maim and KILL!

Autism though is not untreatable. Some NLDs with some patients can be virtually eliminated by removing the cause(s) so the child or adult goes on to live a relatively normal life if it is caught early enough. It is not possible to over-emphasize the VITAL importance of the earliest possible identification for all autistics and NLD people for this and numerous other reasons which we'll consider later. Because of factors like air and water pollution, there has certainly been a dramatic rise in the number of NLD children worldwide over the last 25 to 30 years.

Autism/NLD: What's the difference?

On the face of it there is usually a little apparent difference in outward symptomology between individuals from either group: Anything from mild Dyslexia, to deep, perhaps non-verbal comprehension requiring constant care in all ways. Principally, NLD causes and signs are more often found in various parts of the right side of the brain, although no one is yet sure why or how.

Classical autism in stark contrast is predominantly located in the left and front parts of the brain and is acquired through the parents' germ-lines- and those trends run through families. Thus, when attempting to diagnose either, the specialist must take detailed family history, back to as many generations as possible.

The person's function affected can differ significantly from NLD. This core difference has become much clearer recently, at least in part due to the technical advances in diagnosis we have mentioned. Regrettably, this equipment is far from universally available and a large number of professionals around the world still have to rely on Dr. Kraepelin's Differential Diagnostic method.

As is so often the case in all sciences, there is an unexplained anomaly. That is; a prime Diagnostic presentation for NLD is a substantial gap between Performance IQ and Verbal IQ, the latter being by far higher. That is also the first diagnostic criterion for Asperger's (but NOT for classical autism spectrum disorders). That is very confusing.

Regardless, no practitioner should diagnose from one symptom alone in any situation.

There is though, yet more to Classical Autism: The actual physical and chemical structure, shape and folding patterns of the brain are different from ordinary people; an extra development, especially in the left and frontal lobes of the brain is often found in AS people. This may be where any superior function arises. The left brain is associated with mathematical, logic and language skills, the right side more with spatial perception and art, which will be different from the normal left/right proportions This affects the autistic person's physical, emotional and intellectual reaction and experience of the world. Autistics literally see and feel the world in a totally different way from NTs. That is why they are often said to "be in a world of their own." They are! From this comes the frequent refrain from people that Autistics seem to have a mysterious "otherworldly quality about them," be in "dreamland," or have their "heads in the clouds."

From those with extra right frontal development as well as left, the artistic ability - even genius arises. The clearest examples of how that works in practice may lie in the paintings of the Dutch artists Vincent Van Gogh and Jan Vermeer, both Aspie geniuses with the added ability to paint the world not only as they saw it, but as they felt it.

Naturally from this spatial imbalance we see also one of the roots of Autistic Dyslexia. Another is short-term memory problems, forgetting where they put the car or house keys. One reason for this maybe that their mind is working so fast that it has started on a new task or line of thought before completing and remembering the current one. That is one of many possible explanations of ADD (attention deficit disorder) and ADHD; both of which are associated presentations common to most Dyslexics. The word in the brain is partially forgotten and therefore incomplete before its full message reaches the hand, or the process is reversed, because the brain has moved on to the next word(s) before completing the current one.

Autist Fact: Some Autists repeat, especially when excited the last word(s) of any sentence they are speaking or writing, quite unconsciously, it's another form of verbal "stimming (I do it)."

To sum up: NLD is due to brain differences or damage of varying nature leading to some developmental variances of differing severity and is not present at birth. Classical Autism is due to a different, inherited brain structure, which can result in anything from severe developmental problems to extraordinary abilities and is present from birth but always appears before the age of three. The fact is there is still a great deal about the brain we don't understand. (McWilliams, C W,1999 *Treatment Form Formulary: 6th edition, v*olume 8)

Now that nearly every day new research around the world is shedding increasing light on this complex subject and resolving some of the apparent paradoxes and gaps within the current theories, we can reasonably hope for greater progress and an increasingly better understanding, support and treatments for all forms of Autism and NLDs within the next 5-10 years if more research money and human resources were made available.

There is also another form of NLD that can also cause autism-like behaviors, which to differentiate it, is called NSLD-Non-Specific Learning Difficulty, which has much the same symptoms as autism and NLD, but no agreed cause(s) can be found. Almost everything in this book applies equally to people with an NSLD and to their caregivers/teachers.

Other autism-like conditions:

Williams' Syndrome (WS)

Named after the New Zealander; Dr. Williams who first described it in a 1961 academic paper. It is a very, very rare condition, affecting only about one person in twenty thousand. It is also a very noticeably autistic-like condition, which due to its unique genetic signature is now so well understood by science that it provides convincing evidence of the existence of classical autism as previously described. The cause is that well over twenty genes are simply absent from an area on the seventh Chromosome compared with an average person-leaving the person "incomplete" in their genetic make-up.

The results of Williams' Syndrome are far-reaching and sadly incurable. There are many, but to list a few: Williamsonians have very friendly, outgoing and trusting personalities—like a lot of Autists—but are usually intellectually weak to a greater or lesser degree—along clearly autistic lines—and many cannot live their lives unassisted. Typically, they tend to be shorter and slimmer than the average person. They have characteristically thin, sharply defined, almost pixie or Hobbit-like faces and engaging smiles. Lots of them are especially articulate public and private speakers and charming to know. The majority are very musical, and lots have "perfect pitch" and like many other autistics have an above average tendency to be left-handed, left-footed and left-eye dominant. Virtually all autistics have a special talent of some kind(s), regardless of IQ. Some Williams' people have IQ's of only 60, compared with the average of 100, but they still retain that same lovely, open and warm personality along with their other qualities. It can only be described as "A goodness of spirit" (I. Hale). **Once again this shows how a person's worth cannot and should not be measured solely by their IQ and that message was yet another motivation for writing of this book.**

Perhaps the most obvious physical feature of Williams' Syndrome is that the bridge of the nose starts much lower down the face than is normal. That is also true of Autists, but, in most cases to a less obvious degree.

Sadly, WS also brings with it severe problems with heart function and causes a narrowing of the arteries (termed "Stenosis" by surgeons). Williamsonians are very likely to suffer heart failure and strokes and do not often live a full lifespan. Furthermore, sufferers are prone to over-store calcium, which is in itself dangerous, as it blocks up the cardio -vascular- system-the arteries and veins serving the heart, so they need to avoid Vitamin D3 as it increases calcium retention, and calcium deposits block blood vessels. This and normal arterial calcium build-up (arteriosclerosis) appears to be reversed for ALL people by the right dosage of vitamin K2 (MK-7 variant). Unfortunately, very few doctors know that, and the dosages need to be precise (Vermeer, C 2018).

In a further cruel twist of fate, this means Williams' people are likely to suffer from Multiple Sclerosis (MS)-type symptoms which virtually mirror many of those of Vitamin D3 deficiency. This can lead even experienced doctors to misdiagnose one for the other in anyone.

This happens to ordinary members of the public as well. Always seek a second, and third opinion on MS. It may be just vitamin D3 deficiency in some instances, especially if the patient lives in a low sunlight country. It is notable that a higher percentage of people living in Northern Europe get diagnosed with MS than in sunny Southern Europe. The same applies to parts of America. Anyone living in these areas needs to take the Vitamin supplement, at around 1000 iu per day for an adult or child, says Dr. Michael Holick, MD, Ph. D of Boston University Medical Center. He is the world's leading authority on Vitamin D and its importance, being a professor of Pediatrics, Biophysics and Biochemistry and the author of *The Vitamin D Solution,* 2011.

A 2009 study by Dr. Jodie Barton of the University of Toronto, Canada even found that high doses of Vitamin D dramatically cut the relapse rates among her group of actual MS patients. An interesting rider to this is: a lack of maternal and subsequent embryonic Vitamins and other vital nutrients has been proposed as a cause of Autism, although-to my knowledge- there has been little research into the idea... until governments began to warn people to stay out of the sun in the 1990's for fear of skin cancer-and that naturally Vitamin D3 is made in the skin by the action of sunlight-our collective Vitamin D levels have dropped at about the same time as NLD levels have risen. Of course, correlation doesn't prove cause, but it does ask us some big questions, not least is: "why won't politicians leave medical advice to the professionals".

Note: Vitamin D2 is not the same and much less important, any normal diet provides enough.

As an aside, Vitamin D isn't a vitamin at all, it's a hormone because it's made in a body organ-the skin. That wasn't realized at the time of its discovery in America in 1913, when it was originally synthesized from cod liver oil.

Down's syndrome

Down's syndrome is not an autistic condition, but it does share a few characteristics with some forms of Autism, severe intellectual disability being one and a smaller than average head being another. Downs people like Williamsonians have that fun, charming and loving personality.

That said, Down's syndrome is another piece of the overall picture, in that it too, like Williams Syndrome is a proven genetic condition, the cause of which is a complete or partial third copy of Chromosome 21 (we're only supposed to have two copies of each of our twenty-three pairs of chromosomes). All this aside, knowing Down's people and their carers, they have all said that the advice in this book has been highly useful and relevant to their lives, as well as to Autists. I hoped always to make this piece as inclusive as possible, especially as many of the health, education and social strategies later outlined are equally valid and helpful for NTs as well—of any age or diagnosis.

Autism and Epilepsy: Is there a connection?

Since the late 1960's there have been whispers among groups of teachers, doctors and psychologists that certain "Special Education Needs" (SEN) children, in this instance Autistic pupils, seemed more prone to seizures than other groups. There was no real body of evidence available, just "word of mouth." It is now possible, following a great deal of research from various groups and individuals in recent times and from across the world to reveal the answer.

That answer is now categorically "Yes." About one-in-three Autists experience more than one epileptic seizure during their lifetime. (US National Library/Institutes of Health-PubMed, 2005), other, later studies have confirmed those findings. The average epilepsy rate within the general adult population is about five people per thousand only (WHO). One seizure does not make a person an epileptic, the diagnosis requires at least three or four.

This is in comparison with the rate of three hundred and thirty-four per thousand for Autists. Everyone was sure the two conditions must somehow be linked—but they couldn't find how—and they were right, as was finally proved by the following author's redact of an article published in *ScienceDaily*, April the 8, 2011.

"Researchers have identified a new gene that predisposes people to both autism and epilepsy. The team led by the neurologist Dr. Patrick Cossette, found a severe mutation of the synapsin gene (SYN1-which affects the brain) in all members of a large French-Canadian family suffering from epilepsy, including individuals also suffering from autism. This study includes an analysis of two cohorts of individuals from Quebec, which made it possible to identify other mutations in the SYN1 gene among 1% and 3.5% of those suffering respectively from autism and epilepsy, while several carriers of the SYN1 mutation displayed marked symptoms of both disorders.

"The results show for the first time the role of the SYN1 gene in autism, in addition to epilepsy, and strengthen the hypothesis that a deregulation of the function of synapses because of this mutation is {part of-} the cause of both conditions, until now, no other genetic study of humans has made this demonstration."

Author's note: A Synapse is the brain's equivalent of a postal delivery worker; we have about one thousand TRILLION in our brains, and each directs electrical messages to their proper destination-or not in this and other conditions)

Dr. Cossette also mentioned that this correlation of epilepsy with autism makes the two "co-morbid," which means that if two or more illnesses co-exist at the same time as a normal occurrence, so doctors know there's a connection between them. This is an illuminating piece of research because it irrefutably ties autism-which is broadly but wrongly seen as a purely mental condition-with one that is very obviously purely physical in nature, although both are brain-based. This leads us towards the greater understanding of Autism for what it truly is: a *"Whole Body Condition,"* because our individual genetic profile is written into every cell of our body. For that reason, I advise all autistic/AS patients of all ages to always wear a "Medic Alert" bracelet or lanyard identifying their condition in case of emergency. If cost forbids that, a signed doctor's note with emergency contact details in a plastic card wallet works equally well.

Imagine the sheer wretched hopelessness of having the perceived stigmas of autism AND epilepsy together. To give a sharp perspective on that-it was not until 1970 that epileptics were even allowed to marry in the United Kingdom. In the developing world only one epileptic in ten ever receives treatment, not necessarily because the family is unaware of it or can't afford it, but because it will not admit to the community the "shame" of an epileptic son or daughter, fearing (usually correctly) that it would make all their children unmarriageable.

Add autism to that mix and that's what I meant about "returning the gift."

It is a horrible thing to have to write and to read… but this book deliberately never avoids any controversial or unpleasant matters, in this instance murder. The reality is that in many, probably most countries there are TODAY as yesterday and tomorrow children being murdered by their parents for being "different" in some way: often for being Down's, Autist and/or epileptic, because the family can't or won't deal with the reality of looking after these children and to hide the child's condition from the community. Usually, we see and hear nothing of these murders because they are done at home, in secret. The child is starved or allowed to die of an otherwise easily curable illness. In a few cases, there is a dramatic, violent murder, that makes news headlines—but these are only the tip of a huge global iceberg.

Terminology for the C21st:

Over the years many of us have become increasingly frustrated and dissatisfied with the use of negative and prejudicial terminology about Autism. If we pull together, we can change that perception directly. Let's start with the word "Disorder," again, having its origin in that word Dys/Dis- "bad," a word which has terrible connotations of inferiority and even resonances of malice, then there is "disability" "mental illness" and "defect." Yes, in a substantial number of people autism does reduce their ability to function fully and happily in most societies. That we recognize. However, there are those like Dr. Smith for whom it is a real superpower- not a disability. Therefore, would not the term "Condition" or "State" be both more legitimate and less stigmatizing?

In addition, we should all stop to think…and be very uncomfortable with some of the negative and judgmental terminology used in the fields of medicine, education and psychology both child and adult.

Even if a person's educational potential is greatly limited by one or more of these conditions, we should remember three things: 1) It does not diminish their humanity, 2) It is not their "fault" and 3) Improvement, however great or small is always possible with the right support.

For these reasons, we should consider, and this guide proposes, the abandonment of such terms as NLD and other so-called "disorders," and replacing them with the terms Alternative Education/Employment Profiles (**AEP**s, I. Hale, 2002) with the additional Descriptor of Autistic or Non-Autistic and followed by their characteristics. Then ADHD becomes "an autistic AEP characterized by ……." with the client's name, and assessment. This should automatically generate an Individual Development or Care Program (**I D/CP**) agreed upon between the client, a professional assessor and the carer/advocate as appropriate, regardless of the client's age. It is profoundly damaging, confidence-killing and terrifying to be causally "labelled" and shoved into a convenient and unexplained dark pigeonhole-for life, especially for a child. To have one's cards and future so strongly and adversely marked in advance from such an early age is a fearful experience and a violation of the most basic human rights as well as of the human spirit.

It is also a cruelly overlooked fact that the needs and abilities of autistic adults are all-too-often under-appreciated or ignored altogether, in the family, in society as a whole and in the workplace. Autistic people have a great deal to offer. To waste that potential talent pool may be cheap and convenient to the short-term thinking, small-minded mentality in the areas of education and employment but it is professionally, ethically, financially and morally indefensible. Fortunately, a few employers are now beginning to realize the special talents Autistic people can possess and are actively recruiting them; the German electronics company SAP and Microsoft being two shining but all-too-rare examples. Happily, every day more are following their lead.

This book will continue to use the term HFA, as it will the name AS for Dr. Hans Asperger, who published his seminal paper on the subject in 1944, less than a year after Autism had first been fully described, despite the highly controversial decision of the APA to drop the actual term from its 2013 DSM-5 rewrite.

It has also become clear that the use of the word "spectrum" in this context, although very descriptive and upbeat with its implied relationship to a rainbow is factually misleading, as it conjures up an image of gradation, that is, of each component lying neatly next to its neighbor like the tools laid out on a carpenter's bench or items on a store shelf. As we have seen, all the types of autism/AS are overlapping and intersecting in complex ways and at the deepest levels and never found in isolation, whether they are Classical or non-Classical in origin.

For this reason, let us replace "The Autistic Spectrum" with "The Autism family tree," illustrated below as a much more representative scientific and practical description of this complex subject, showing how autism comes in so many varieties and combinations, as well as how every part is inseparable from the rest.

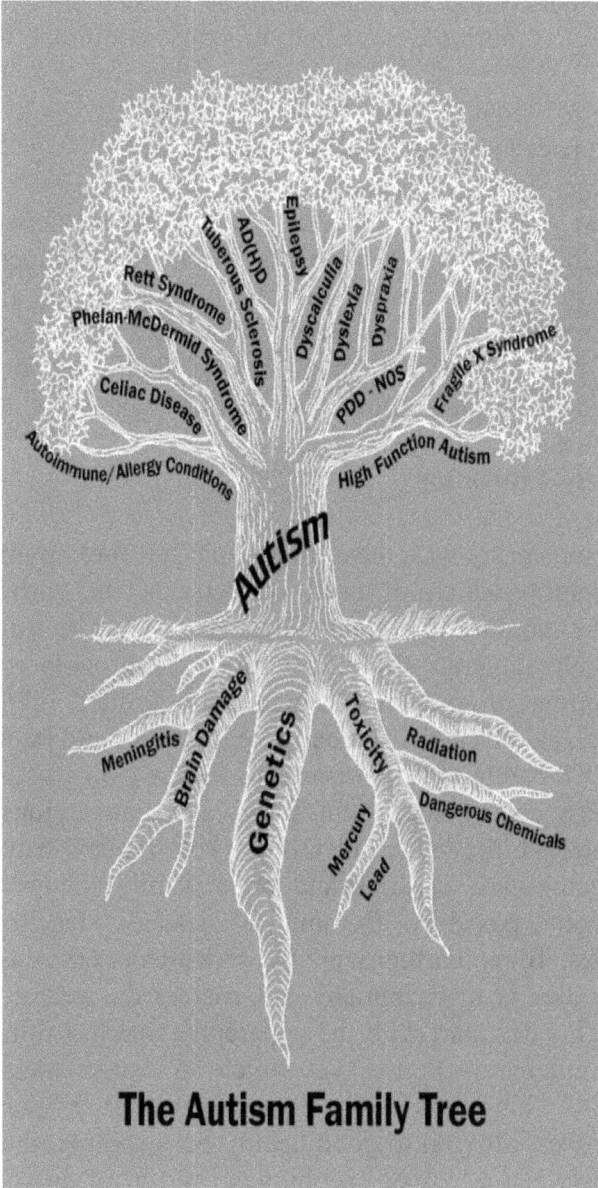

The Autism family tree by Prof. David P Burkart

Here are the principal conditions, sub-conditions, related branches and some of the co-morbidities which together comprise the Autism Family.

They include Epilepsy, Tuberous sclerosis, and dyslexia.

A Few Fun Facts: Autistic/AS Comedians, actors and musicians: Dan Ackroyd ("Ghostbusters," "The Blues Brothers"), Eminem, Gary Numan, Marty Balin (Jefferson Airplane), John Denver, Jim Henson (The Muppets), singer/songwriter, James Taylor, John Lennon and further back and significantly, both classical composers, Wolfgang Amadeus Mozart, and Gustav Mahler.

Autism and Society-Education:

All autistic conditions bring with them an unusual gift for copying, memory and imitation which, if used correctly at the earliest possible age can be turned into a real advantage. The key to using that capacity to help integrate the Autist more comfortably into society is the finding of and encouragement to imitate highly positive role models. Conversely, if a bad role model should be the only one available, it can be doubly disastrous for the over-trusting Autist. This strategy can be successful at any age, but obviously the younger it's started, the better. Ideally the role models would be the parents, caregivers, siblings and other family members. Where that is not possible, Community leaders, teachers, characters in books, films, cartoons or TV series can serve very well instead. The idea is to encourage- not coerce- the Autist to copy the model. This can start with the apparently simplest things which an NT would barely notice, yet which an Autist doesn't understand at all: Things like dental and personal hygiene, showers, clean clothes, all vital to good health. For example, there is a proven link between a lack of oral hygiene and heart disease- and to social comfort.

Autists aren't slovenly, but they can at times be oblivious to themselves and others. Hair care and nails are other often overlooked areas. Social manners too can be taught using this method, "please" "thank you," "excuse me" "how are you"? "Would you like something to eat/drink," "well done," shaking hands, learning to look people in the eye, making small talk, all the little things; the social give-and-take (reciprocity) and politeness that make up the everyday workings of any society and which are essential for a successful and happy life in the NT world. The same is true of dress codes; what-to-wear at certain events; job interviews are an important example. As the Autist masters these foundation skills, more and more skills and nuances can be added. This process may seem trivial to some, but I and others have found it really helpful. It adds up over the years and produces profound rewards even though it takes a long time-and a lot of trial and error. Patience coupled with determination is the key to success.

Chapter 5: The Main Roots and Theories of Autism and NLDs

As we now understand Autism is a long-established collection of a sufficient number of specific behaviors, the syndromes of which may be produced by one or more of the stimuli we'll examine in this chapter.

Firstly, TBIs as doctors call them—Traumatic Brain Injuries—a big whack on the head to the rest of us. :) They can be caused by direct blows or by being hit by a pressure wave following an explosion in one form or another. Either can result in permanent physical damage to the brain. If the damaged areas are the ones which relate to autism, that person will become autistic, if to a different area, the person will become NLD.

Secondly, certain diseases: There are four basic categories of disease that can directly damage the brain like TBIs.

The most common is Meningitis- an infection of the protective membrane that encloses the brain and spine and is usually caused by one of any number of different bacteria, although there are viral types as well.

Encephalitis is anything that causes the brain itself to swell and become damaged, it is usually caused by some virus or other, Rubella is one of those as is CMV (Cytomegalovirus), one of the Herpes family, as are "cold sores." Rubella is better known as "German Measles" and can be life-threatening to young children. There are very effective vaccines against all of the above and my strong advice to any parent is to have your child vaccinated against them as early as possible.

The third category are the degenerative brain conditions, caused by the brain or its blood supply becoming clogged up, usually by plaque deposits and/or knot-like protein tangles of various descriptions which disrupt the brain's function. These result in parts of the brain dying over time. Parkinson's disease (PD) and Alzheimer's disease (AD) are two and vary only by where in the brain the plaquing occurs, as they both produce much the same tragic effects of which we're all well aware. The loss of memory, sense of smell, mobility, personality changes, speech difficulty and loss of personal and spatial awareness, among others. During the phases of both these and related conditions, strongly autistic traits can be noticed.

Aluminum ingestion has been linked to Alzheimer's. Research published in the *Journal of Applied Toxicology,* indicated long-term exposure to human mammary (Breast) epithelial cells contaminated with aluminum can in some incidences result in anchorage-independent growth, a key indicator of cultured tumor cells (cancer) and of cells on the way to becoming malignant. This is still not proven conclusively. A widely used product containing aluminum is underarm deodorant; aluminum is quickly absorbed into the body through the skin. There are many others; cake mix and some suntan products being just two, again emphasizing the other hazards of toxic metals, aside from Autism. To be safe, try to avoid metal products, especially when pregnant and/or breastfeeding.

Similarly, the same Autistic presentation may happen with cerebral arteriosclerosis (CA). With this the arteries and capillaries supplying blood and oxygen to the head become increasingly narrowed and hardened by deposits and age and again, those parts of the brain affected, begin to wither and then stop working. If those parts are the ones which, when affected, are the ones which produce autism or NLD these conditions will appear.

Fourthly, if the blockages in the blood circulatory system occur to the brain spontaneously, these are known as Strokes. If they occur in the lungs, Pulmonary Embolisms; and if in the heart, Heart Attacks or "Cardio-vascular events." In each event brain damage may result from lack of oxygen being supplied to the brain (Hypoxia).

The general perception of these degenerative conditions is that they only affect the seniors' age group, which WAS generally true. Today though, we are increasingly seeing them: PD, AD and CA in the age 35-40 group and that is also true of heart disease.

Premature Birth and Low Birth weight: Studies in 2008 by the famous McGill Medical School in Montreal, Canada found that babies born seven to fourteen weeks too early were four times more likely to exhibit signs of autism/NLD. In 2011 a team from Pennsylvania led by Jennifer Pinto-Martin studied nearly a thousand early—born of low weight and found they were up to five times more likely to be autistic than the average, probably due to the brain having insufficient time to fully develop. This research though begs an unanswered question… namely-were these children born too early because they had inherited autism at conception, or did their premature birth cause their autism?

Finally, cancer (and some chemo-therapy cancer drugs) can damage the brain and may lead to NLDs presenting at any stage of life.

Environmental:

In this section we are looking at environmental agents that can cause brain damage and lead to NLDs, usually from birth or in young children. This whole question is under-researched, and few authorities seem to actually want to conduct thorough large-scale studies, perhaps due to the pressure from corporate or industrial lobbying groups? The word for these substances is "Teratogens" and refers to any materials that can cause multiple birth and growth defects in people, other animals and plants. Among well-known ones are excessive exposure to many types of pesticides, herbicides (weed killers) and radiation to the mother, father and/or fetus.

Horrifying evidence for this has emerged from the cities in Japan which were nuclear bombed in 1945; Hiroshima and Nagasaki, where radiation-caused birth defects continue to stalk each new generation to this day, autism included. The lands surrounding the shattered nuclear power plant at Chernobyl in the Ukraine are another high-profile example. There is also cursory and anecdotal evidence that children born near old, leaky nuclear power plants and other installations, such as Sellafield, in Cumbria County in the United Kingdom, as well as chemical factories also suffer far higher levels of cancer and other health-related problems compared with the national average—and the existence of "childhood cancer clusters" is well recorded and accepted by many people around the world.

Those industries affect the plant and animal life around them as well, whether by land, sea, air or in nearby rivers. The results are clearly visible in birth deformities to the wildlife, which, along with the local water supply, finds its way up the food chain into our shops and bodies. Very similar patterns of child deformity and adult sickness are still found in Vietnam, Laos and Cambodia after the use of the defoliant chemical spray "Agent Orange" during the Vietnam War to destroy tree cover.

Diabetes during pregnancy, as well as high alcohol consumption can cause birth abnormalities of numerous types, as of course can tobacco smoking. Some High Fructose Corn Syrups (HFCS) have been suggested to be harmful. So far, the clinical evidence for that has proved inconclusive. Proven Teratogens though include certain Organophosphate-based products including household cleaners, food additives, pesticides and weed killers such as Roundup (now banned in many countries) as shown by various studies conducted in 2005 and then by the California Department of Public Health in 2007. Adding more weight to the environmental causes, a survey conducted in 2011 suggests living near the fumes of a main road may damage the baby's development.

Many common items now contain Organophosphates, especially furniture because they're effective fire resisters.

The horrendous effects on every area of the human and all other animals' body (heart, brain, cancer, etc.) at any age due to the ingestion of numerous micro-plastics is well proven, but the full long-term whole planetary extent and seriousness is still part of continuing research including: https://hph.stanford.edu/focal_areas/pollution_health/plastics-and-health-working-group

My advice is to boil all drinking water (filters aren't fine enough), avoid cooking in plastic containers, avoid tinned foods, and do not eat or drink from plastic containers.

Increasing female obesity in the Western world—being too fat—has also been shown to predispose children to autism (*Pediatrics*: April 9, 2012).

There are other theories; including low maternal thyroid function, causing a lack or overdose of the hormone, Thyroxine.

All pregnant women should get a thyroid test as early in the pregnancy as possible for their own sake as well as baby's. High household stress or depression levels, which abnormally raise levels of the hormone Cortisol (The Stress Hormone) perhaps from financial hardship seem to cause babies of below average weight to be born, but any connection to that or thyroid levels with autism/AS, is still tentative, as is another very new theory. The theory suggests older fathers (defined as being over forty) are more likely to have autistic or schizophrenic offspring than those of younger ones. This is only though according to a single study conducted by a team in Iceland and using a very small sample of only eighty-eight children.

Pre-natal exposure to some prescription medicines, as well as illegal street drugs such as solvents, Meth, Crack, PCP (phenylcyclohexylpiperidine) and heroin are well known to damage the developing child. A class of chemicals called BPAs, Bis phenol-A which seeps out of common plastic bags and bottles, is regarded by many scientists to be a serious danger, with strong evidence to back up that claim, including an in-depth study published in The *Journal of Human Reproduction*, July 31, 2013, linking them with falling human fertility rates (and by extension, that of other creatures).

The same has been found of other forms of Organophosphate as well as PCBs-Polychlorinated biphenyls, used in a wide variety of products from paints to adhesives to lubricating agents and some common household electrical devices. There is an increasing body of evidence that ironizing EMR (Electro-magnetic radiation) can cause cancer anywhere in the body, at any age including the brain. EMR has been directly blamed for the perceived rise in autism since the 1970's as our exposure to it (in the industrialized world) has increased more than sixty-times since then. EMR emitters embrace pretty much anything electrical, Televisions, hairdryers, microwave ovens, cellular phones and thousands more items. Living near cell phone masts, electricity sub-stations or high-voltage power lines would also greatly increase the exposure level and many people who live close to these sources report serious health problems from across the world. Children are especially vulnerable to these effects as it affects their normal growth.

There has simply not been enough research to either fully confirm or refute these ideas...but it is worth noting that in April 2011 the WHO issued a strong warning that hand-held mobile phones are linked to a certain type of brain cancer-Glioma (from which Senator Edward Kennedy died) – based mainly on a study by their International Agency for Research on Cancer (IARC) led by Dr. Jonathon Samet of the University of Southern California and on findings from the 1960's onwards conducted in Sweden. That research is ongoing and is increasingly disturbing in its implications as the data mounts up concerning over-use of mobile telephones and other mobile devices. The effects of the new 5G system have yet to be studied, but their potential danger should cause us real concern, because the numerous "booster stations" needed to make the system work will expose many more people to ironizing radiation-the most dangerous type regarding cancer and abnormal childhood development. Radiation affects DNA and therefore, everything we are.

Toxicity—poisons:

Firstly, lots of poisons from household products (e.g. dishwasher fluid, floor polish, and some soaps) can damage the body and brain. Rat poison, carbon monoxide gas, arsenic, and perhaps in the case of both children and adults excess mono-sodium-glutamate (MSG) in food (it's an additive which boosts taste) and is considered by many to be harmful, although the evidence is sketchy so far.

Aspartame is a clear danger. It's an artificial sweetener whose appalling side-effects have been widely posted since the 1990's. Yet along with high-energy, high-sugar drinks which have been linked to both ADHD-type symptoms and certain cancers it is still available in confectionaries, drinks and numerous other products on every store shelf (*American Journal of Clinical Medicine,* December 2012). Other rare but possible culprits are a few types of mold and fungi which are known to cause brain damage, fungal meningitis being one.

NIDS: Is a new theory: it is Neuro-Immune Dysfunction Syndrome. The theory is that the autism traits are a by-product of a weakened immune system stemming from a single continuous and perhaps almost unnoticeable (asymptomatic, meaning there are no clearly visible symptoms, like a fever) low-level attack, normally by a virus. Again, this is unproven, but it's always worth getting a broad series of viral tests, as at least some can be cured.

This wide range of tests is a "Viral Panel." What is sure is that some viruses cause cancer. Hepatitis strains can cause liver cancer, as can about thirty of the hundreds of strains of the Human Papillomavirus (HPV), a common sexually transmitted virus affecting up to eight out of ten British adults and about twenty million Americans. It has been shown to produce a variety of throat and reproductive system cancers, including cervical, penile and mouth. It can be carried and transmitted by both genders. In

2008 the United Kingdom began a vaccination program targeting girls between the ages of twelve and thirteen. Time has shown this was a very good idea because it has cut infection rates dramatically. Still, why not target boys equally, that smacks of gender discrimination to me. HPV is part of the same virus family as Cytomegalovirus (CMV) and the Epstein-Barr Virus (EBV) causing Mononucleosis/Glandular Fever, both of which may be among the causes of various cancers.

A virus can cause cancer by inhabiting and altering the genetic structure of every cell of your body, including brain cells, in doing so they cause a genetic mutation in some cells, which can then become malignant.

This genetic hijacking is the basis of another theory: that autism/NLD is the result of viral infections affecting the brain structure, either before birth or shortly afterwards- before the child's immune system is well developed. Once again, this is an interesting and logical idea and one which ties in well with the NIDS theory, but both remain under-researched, so we can't yet be positive one way or the other, more research is needed.

Lastly the increasingly well researched and funded work done by Professor Simon Baron-Cohen (Oscar-winning comedian Ali G's cousin), head of the Autism Research Centre (ARC) and his team at England's prestigious Cambridge University and arguably the world's leading authority on Asperger's Syndrome. This involves the pre-birth environment- of the baby (Fetus) in the mother's womb (Uterus). He calls it the FT (Fetal Testosterone) theory. Broadly, he has found that some babies are exposed to higher testosterone levels in the womb than others. (Testosterone is the main male hormone, but all women have a small amount naturally). It seems that a few women have at times unusually high levels which affect the baby, giving it (male or female) in some areas markedly stronger (Traditionally) masculine traits, specifically with regards to a perceived lack of emotional and social empathy and reciprocity, which are very Aspie characteristics.

Professor Baron-Cohen controversially believes **this** is what AS actually is, and some of his supporters believe that it further applies, in different degrees, to other members of the autism family, notably PDD-NOS. It is broadly referred to as the "Extreme Male Brain Theory." It does not mean that such people have a brutish "Caveman Complex," far from it, but it may explain at least one aspect of the mystery of the severe social disability which Asperger's Syndrome certainly is.

It is an immensely complex bio-chemical and psychological work that is well beyond the scope of this book to detail in its entirety. Research into it continues. From it, Baron-Cohen has evolved his "Empathy-Systematizing Theory," which we'll explore later.

Autie/AS Myth bites the dust. Surprisingly, a lot of people share the belief that Autists in general and Aspies in particular are unable to lie or detect sarcasm and irony. That isn't at all true, except during childhood. We can lie, or at least we sometimes edit the full truth, as part of the "masking" strategy we have discussed. We can also bluff very convincingly, aided by our tendency to have expressionless faces. A tip-never play poker against a skilled Aspie unless you have lots of money to lose. :)

What is true is that we are very literal, that is; we take words and actions entirely at face-value because we cannot understand social or vocal cues, hints, flirting or nuances. Please just say what you mean! We also tend to respond in a very straight-forward, perhaps one-dimensional manner, so yes, we are by nature very honest and straight-talking. That is another personality trait which is frequently misunderstood and interpreted as hostile or rude. We're not good at shallow flattery or "small talk." Some people find that honesty refreshing, more seem to find it offensive or just unsettling, which, not having those social skills Aspies simply can't understand any more than they can understand the consequences of their words to the point if/until they learn to self-censor, or "mask"- in public at least.

The constant rebuffs resulting from this directness only add to the Autist's sense of alienation from mainstream society and increase their withdrawal and "closed-in-ness," a classic viscous circle. That said, life experience of the NT world quickly teaches us to dissemble or lie when we must-it doesn't come naturally... but it does come eventually as a self-defense tactic and social self-censoring can be taught successfully using the techniques in this book. Hmmm, think before you speak or act about how the other person might receive or respond to what you say or do.

True story: A friend (Aspies do have them, just not very many) asked me about a prescription-only medicine "Where did you find it"? To which I replied (not trying to be sarcastic), "at the chemist." That's how literal Aspies are.

Chapter 6: The Dangers of Metals, Fluoride, and the Word on Vaccines

This section's main focus is on heavy metal poisoning. Almost all metals when swallowed, inhaled or absorbed through the skin are dangerous, among the worst are Silver, Aluminum -the recommendation is not to cook in (or drink from) uncoated Aluminum pots, foil or pans (Global Health Center) - Gold, Beryllium, Tin, Lead, Copper, Arsenic, Cadmium, Mercury, Nickel and Zinc, although zinc in small amounts-about 10 mg a day is vital for a strong immune system.

Generally, the heavier and softer the metal, the more and quicker the damage it does. So, we shall focus mainly on Lead, Mercury, Gold and Copper, four very common metals, each with well-proven links to autism. In all cases the amounts needed to cause serious harm can arrive suddenly in an accident or accumulate over time.

A note on Gold: The ancient tradition of a trader biting a coin or token offered by a stranger has its basis in it being soft. There will be a bite mark left on a genuine gold piece; no mark showed that the piece was a painted iron fake. Gold is also a toxic metal if ingested in Sulphate form as a treatment for rheumatism (in some cultures).

Copper: Probably the least reported but most common form of heavy metal poisoning. Excess copper comes from many sources, copper piping for household or industrial water supplies, copper cooking utensils, it is in virtually every electrical device and being a soft, malleable metal like gold, is easily absorbed through the skin over extended periods. It is doubly dangerous to children, who naturally put virtually anything in their mouths to suck, chew or eat. Copper is also readily absorbed from copper bracelets and other jewelry. We can get it in high amounts from red meat, wheat, nuts, all shellfish, coffee, chocolate and green-leaf vegetables like lettuce and from mushrooms.

Physically, a liver disorder as well as excess from these sources can lead to the build-up of copper in the body known as "Copper Toxicity Syndrome," (CTS) as the liver is the organ which stores and regulates copper levels. The right amount of copper is good, it promotes protein absorption, efficient energy production and healthy bones, but too much, detected by a hair, blood or eye test is very harmful. An inherited condition in which the liver stores excess copper instead of excreting it is named Wilson's disease and in its later stages can be diagnosed by an eye examination, from the distinctive copper-colored rings-Kaiser-Fleischer rings- around the Iris of the eye. This can be successfully treated in a number of ways, drugs or Chelation being the usual ones.

Excess copper is known to be a causal factor and/or a trigger for autism, Alzheimer's, bi-polar disorder (originally known as Manic-Depression) schizophrenia, Chronic Fatigue Syndrome (CFS) loss of mobility, hallucinations, low immune function, loss of social function-the person gradually becomes more withdrawn-another autistic trait- liver disease, ADD, ADHD, ME (Myalgic Encephalomyelitis) adrenal malfunction, depression, muscle withering and many more. It can also trigger anorexia. The point is that CTS appears to be a purely psychological condition, whereas it's a physical one- it takes a very good doctor to spot that. There is even a typical "Copper Toxicity Syndrome" personality; warm, caring, lovable, outgoing-very much like Williams' sufferers. If, like gold poisoning, it is left untreated, it is fatal, they all are.

If you ever suspect anyone in the family of having CTS, get a hair test. If the adult level is above 25 ppm (parts per million) see a specialist and change your lifestyle. For children, this is even more vital, as they can suffer permanent brain and Central Nervous System (CNS) damage. The CNS controls every function of the body. It is frightening how many CTS and Wilson's sufferers have and still do end up in psychiatric institutions because nobody did one standard simple and inexpensive test.

Excess Tin has long been linked to some lung and eye conditions.

Fluoride: On the third of August 2012 Harvard University's School of Public Health published their findings of a study comprised of 27 research projects over a twenty-two-year period, funded by The Federal National Institutes for Health (NIH) on the effects of large (and it must be stressed, Large) concentrations of Fluoride in the public water supply on developing children. It concluded that virtually worldwide it significantly lowers IQ to a point of making children learning disabled compared with children whose exposure to Fluoride was low or nil.

Lead: Ironically it was copper that replaced Lead as the water piping of choice in the industrialized world. At one time it was used in paint and Pewter for plates and other household utensils, batteries, children's toys, fishing weights and cosmetics in some countries and it is still found everywhere in abandoned industrial sites. Its dangers cannot be overstated. Generally, lead builds up in the body over the years, either through the mouth, eyes, nose or skin.

The results, especially in children, are both horrific and profound and can be fatal. They include a loss of memory, the full range of NLDs, mania/dementia, extreme swings of mood as well as more obviously physical symptoms. These include stomach pain, rashes and severe headaches. Treatment is effective if it's started quickly and is by Chelation therapy, the longer the delay in detecting and treating Lead poisoning the worse the permanent damage will be.

During the eighteenth and nineteenth centuries—the hay-day of the traditional hat-making industry—Lead was used to stiffen, add weight and hold the shape of the hat. The workers—who handled the lead oxide powder all the time—became sick that gave rise to the expression "as mad as a Hatter."

A quick mention of Iron: Over-use of iron supplements or too much iron from another source causes damage to the liver, heart and brain. After the Iron is no longer being taken, recovery is usually pretty rapid with few if any complications in most cases.

The exception is a rare genetic condition called Hemochromatosis, in which the liver stores Iron rather than regulating its level in the body by excreting any excess. Again, it is treated with Chelation and perhaps dialysis if the kidneys are damaged. With prompt treatment most people recover well.

Finally, and perhaps the most dangerous of all, is Mercury, also known as "Quicksilver" on account of its color and the fact that it is the only common metal that is liquid at room temperature or in the sea, making exposure very easy. That adds to its danger. Its highly destructive effects on the liver, kidneys, skin, and brain have all been well documented for decades. It can enter the body in numerous ways: Oily fish such as Salmon and Tuna store Mercury from the sea in their bodies. Some come from natural Mercury ores in the oceans and some from the appalling levels of Industrial effluent dumping.

The same applies to shellfish, especially clams and shrimp. It is in many clinical thermometers (although, due to the danger to patients—especially children—biting them, these are being phased out in favor of alcohol or electronic versions). Barometers, light bulbs (the worst of all being the "energy-savers"), some dyes, amalgam dental fillings—which have now been banned in advanced countries like Germany since the early 1990's—to be replaced by safer, ceramic materials. I advise the replacement, if possible, of all dental amalgam fillings, a mix of Mercury, Silver, Tin and Copper, to all adult clients, not only to help safeguard against autism, but on general health grounds as well. Children should never be given amalgam fillings.

Mercury as heated vapor become airborne from industrial processes including mining and agricultural use and in hospitals, because like Copper it kills germs and fungi very efficiently. There are dozens of other sources too numerous to mention here. There is no longer any reasonable doubt that sufficient Mercury exposure can and does cause autism, most obviously AuDHD by brain and immune system damage at any age. Further studies by America's renowned Harvard University, the CDC (Centers for Disease

Control and Prevention), and the FDA (Food and Drug Administration) going back years confirm all those findings. If you believe there is any chance that you or your child have become affected by metals, please go to a clinic and get tested immediately.

There is also the much talked-about use of mercury compounds in common vaccines, most notoriously the MMR jab (Mumps, Measles, and Rubella). It is used in the form Ethyl Mercury-named Thimerosal as a vital preservative allowing the vaccine to "keep" for long periods, enabling them to be more widely available, especially for transportation to desperate countries in the Developing world. Mercury compounds have been used in scores of vaccines since the 1930's as it still is today, for example in the HPV, Yellow Fever, Polio, Hepatitis B, and Anthrax shots. Regrettably it is still the best preservative we have to date. There is no viable alternative clinically or financially. If we want to keep helping mass populations around the world avoid the plagues of the past, it is not only a clinical necessity but a moral imperative.

The English Controversy:

In 1998 a team of researchers in London led by a Dr. Andrew Wakefield published a report in *The Lancet* journal of medicine linking the MMR vaccine (and citing the Mercury in it) as the cause of both severe gut problems and autism in babies given the jab. Shortly afterwards, having read the article, most of his team disowned it as flawed, incompetent, faked, inadequately evidenced, unethical, and unduly influenced by Wakefield's desire for financial gain. In fact, only twelve carefully selected, already very sick children had been hand-picked by Wakefield for his study and there were no proper comparative (control) peer groups used to establish baseline results. That is, the expected norm, drawn from healthy children who had received the same vaccines at the same age and from a group of those who had not. Worse still, it emerged slowly that Wakefield's children had been seriously assaulted by being given painful, dangerous, and completely unnecessary medical tests and drugs without proper parental consent. Parents had either not been informed at all or lied to later.

Despite numerous attempts by teams round the world, Wakefield's results have never been repeated because they were faked and a fraud from the beginning. In 2004 the highly respected *Sunday Times* journalist, Brian Deer investigated the whole squalid affair including Wakefield's many underhand business dealings and associations.

He published his article and handed the files over to the British medical authorities in the shape of the General Medical Council (GMC) who then belatedly conducted their own investigation. Their report released in 2010 completely discredited Wakefield along with his report and culminated with him being struck off the medical registers of both Britain and the US. He is no longer a Doctor of Medicine.

Meanwhile, the mistaken credibility that Wakefield had achieved by being published in such an established and prestigious British medical journal caused worried parents around the world to withdraw permission for their children to be vaccinated. Over the last fourteen years Britain, Nigeria and other countries, notably in Eastern Europe, Italy, and the USA have witnessed ongoing and growing epidemics of Mumps, Measles, and Rubella, causing some children to die and many more to become permanently severely disabled.

10 very good reasons to vaccinate yourself and your children:

(1) Drug companies and their shareholders know that killing, maiming or poisoning their customers, children, pets, or livestock is bad for business. That's why they spend billions of US dollars on the best laboratories, scientists, and equipment available. To give one example: the best White Laser microscopes in the world are made by Siemens. AG—a personal opinion, but one based on laboratory experience—and cost upwards of six hundred thousand dollars for the base scope alone. Their research costs are

astronomical and the patents last only fifteen years before some "bucket-shop lab" can copy the original formula and make a cheaper but vastly inferior product with untested low-grade ingredients, some of which can be toxic and cause very serious damage to young children and even adults. It is largely THOSE knockoffs which do damage, not reputable ones, and which cause just concerns, both for parents and the medical profession.

No doctor would deny the risks of any low-quality "generic" medicine, just as there are real dangers in low quality contaminated food or water. Anything made by those companies can be dangerous. That is why big drug companies are forced to charge high prices; to finance future high-quality research. In my opinion international drug patent law should be changed to twenty-five or even thirty years. Doing so would allow the drugs to be cheaper as the original companies would have a longer period to recoup their development costs, while better protecting the public from dangerous, imitation drugs.

The following are the tests of good vaccines vs. dangerous ones. (I. Hale, 2025).

Good vaccines are:

a) The formula is carefully worked out, tested in computer simulations, then animal cells in a fully transparent manner.

b) Phases 1-3 of human trials are large mixed randomized groups of 10s of thousands. Again, the results are published.

c) The trials are Double blind with Control groups at each phase.

d) After official, independent certification, the vaccine is manufactured to the highest standards, with the highest quality components and public, regular quality controlled tested. A beacon company is the French Pasteur-Sanofi one.

A safe vaccine should take at least 10 years to develop from concept to use.

Do your research, insist on high quality vaccines.

(2) Autism/AS along with its associated gut conditions like Crohn's and Celiac disease existed well before the 1930's – or vaccines at all. We know this from seeing their characteristic DNA sequences in people from hundreds and thousands of years ago. The DNA sample is taken from teeth or bones by a forensic archaeologist then decoded and examined by a specialist doctor.

Children of my generation were often vaccinated later than now, usually not before first school between the ages of 5 and 8— Classical autism shows before then. This proves that vaccines can't logically be a cause of autism or AS.

(3) Vaccination works: Polio vaccine for example cuts infection levels consistently by over ninety percent worldwide and reduces the severity of the illness for the minority who do still get it even after vaccination. The huge reward vastly outweighs the small risk involved (*Discover*, January 5, 2012)

(4) Vaccination protects not only the vaccinated, but by cutting infection rates reduces disease even among the unvaccinated. This protects the whole community by reducing suffering and time lost at work or school while easing the strain on local and national health services. It is the socially responsible thing to do.

(5) We vaccinate our pets, so why not our children and ourselves? Pet vaccine contains the same trace Mercury preservatives, and I've yet to meet an autistic goldfish or rabbit.

(6) The Ethyl-Mercury compound, Thimerosal—having been in use since 1928—has, after the Wakefield furor, been widely replaced in children's vaccines, although doing so has reduced their strength and shelf-life. It is still used for adult vaccinations. There

has been no corresponding drop-off rate reported in Childhood Autism since then and despite yet another WHO report confirming its safety, for whatever reason some people still refuse to vaccinate. The fact is the amount of mercury in vaccine, compared with that released from a lifetime of amalgam tooth fillings, eating sea foods or getting the much more dangerous purer form, Methyl-Mercury in your body by accident is miniscule and is cleared out by the liver in a few weeks. It takes a big exposure to cause serious harm.

(7) It is worth noting...children are given the MMR shot at eleven months—exactly the "crawling around putting things in their mouth" stage—the discovery of the world outside themselves. If Mercury, or any other damaging contaminate enters them, vaccination is just about the least likely source. There may be an MMR booster shot given to a child at age four, but it isn't always needed and very few concerns have ever been reported during the thirty years it has been in widespread use.

(8) Not all vaccines even contain Mercury these days; the flu vaccine made by the famous Pasteur Institute in France is just one example. If you have concerns, ask for a Mercury-free product. Anyway, have the darn jab!

(9) Talking of flu, you are far more likely to get Guillain-Barre Syndrome (a very rare and serious neurological condition) by having the flu than by having the jab—about forty to seventy times more likely (WHO).

(10) If the current take-up rate of common vaccinations about which we've known since their initial discovery by Edward Jenner in 1796 drops substantially, not only will the great plagues of the past such as Cholera, Polio Typhoid, and Diphtheria return, but there would be no money and therefore no research facilities left to develop new vaccines or cures against current and future plagues, HIV being one. This would leave humanity open to possible catastrophe, as happened with The Black Death in the fourteenth century and who knows, maybe worse in the future? Each jab is an

investment in your children's future, your grandchildren's future, and that of the human race.

And…if vaccines really do cause autism, how come so few vaccinated children actually are autistic?

Advice for Jabs:

If you still have worries, there are a few easy steps you can take to further minimize any risk. MY advice is simple. Give yourself and your children the vaccinations, but spaced separately, 2-4 weeks apart, to allow for full immune system recovery. Yes; Jabs/Shots/Vaccinations, whichever is your preferred term do come with certain occasional risks of which we should be aware to take the necessary precautions, so should your Doctor.

The younger or frailer the patient the greater the risk is, although it is still tiny. Firstly, one person in a few hundred may suffer a marked reaction, such as a rash, soreness, redness/swelling where the shot was given or sleepiness, it needs no treatment and will be fine in a few hours or days, with rest and plenty of water.

In extremely rare cases the reaction can be a violent and perhaps even life threatening (why don't they call it "death-threatening")? This natural allergic reaction is termed "anaphylactic shock" from some trace substance in the vaccine, as some unfortunate people get from common foods such as peanuts.

The shock can be nearly instant or develop over five to ten minutes, which is why it is always wise to sit down for a while in the Doctor's surgery after a shot, just in case. In anaphylactic shock, the person goes into seizure and spasms, their air passages may swell up, causing choking, and there may be cardiac arrest (heart stoppage).

If that happens, the doctor will first administer epinephrine—a stimulant, using an "epipen," a spring-loaded syringe that delivers the shot immediately into a person's thigh muscle and oxygen.

He/she may then use CPR (cardiopulmonary resuscitation) to re-start the heart and lungs if needed or perhaps a defibrillator to deliver an electric shock to re-start the heart. Most patients recover very quickly and are fine. Patients with known serious allergies should always carry an epipen around with them at all times; my Father carried one for wasp and hornet stings.

Secondly, especially for young children; check your child's temperature for fever for the five days before the vaccination appointment and on the day.

The Doctor should do the same (and for adults as well) but not all do. If the person is sick, postpone the date. Vaccinations DO put extra short-term strain on the immune system and if it's already fighting something else a jab can, in very rare instances "crash" it, with serious, perhaps long-term consequences. If you are in any doubt, put off the appointment. For the same reason, take it easy for a few days after the jab. It should be making your immune system work harder to produce the antibodies to protect you from the disease for which the vaccine was given. Afterwards, drink plenty of water, add extra vitamins C & D, get extra rest and of course, you may feel mild symptoms of whatever you've been vaccinated against—that's normal. If you still feel off-color after four days, see a nurse or pharmacist.

Facts on Vaccination: If vaxxing truly caused autism, all vaccinated children would become autistic. **They don't,** again proving there is no link between safe vaxxing and Autism.

The first mass-vaccination program was conducted by Napoleon Bonaparte for his Grand Army in 1805. It was so successful that he ordered the program to be expanded to inoculate the whole of the French people in 1806 with such success that Bavaria and Hesse followed suit in 1807 and Denmark in 1810. No autism epidemic followed any of these initiatives in any country.

Chelation:

In the previous section, "chelation" was used a lot in describing an effective way of treating heavy metal and toxic exposure, so here's how it works-and how it ties in with Autism. The word comes from the same Greek root as Chemistry and refers to the use of chemicals. In this therapy they are known as "Chelating agents" or "Chelators" of which there are many, each one used according to the toxin it is intended to remove.

Chelation therapy goes way back to the Second World War where the first, called "British Anti Lewisite" (BAL) was invented in Oxford to combat the expected use by Germany of Lewisite—a spectacularly nasty Organo-arsenic gas-which in fact never existed. BAL did though prove an effective treatment for removing most heavy metals and poisonous minerals including sulfur from an affected person. It was discovered in 1940 but not declassified for public use until 1945. It is still used today, largely to treat Wilson's disease and Lead poisoning. BAL's chemical name is Dimercaprol.

Normally Chelators are put into the patient as a solution through a tube into an arm vein; this is the IV (Intravenous) method. Like most Chelators BAL has an oily feel to it. BAL though is injected by syringe, painfully, into large muscles. Chelators act by gluing themselves to the toxin, helping to break it up and making it slippery—allowing the body to move it away from regions of accumulation like the liver and into the body's normal systems until it can be excreted naturally via the kidneys. You drink lots of water to basically remove the toxin through the urine. It requires lots of injections and has some nasty side effects.

Among those side effects: and this is true of any chelating agent is that it removes good things as well as bad, such as vitamins, minerals and other nutrients, so supplementing is important during treatment. BAL also causes vomiting, cramps, bone weakness, eye problems—it takes out the semi-fluid in the eye, causing (sometimes) blindness, but most seriously it raises blood pressure very high, very quickly, which can cause fatal hemorrhaging in any major organ in your body. Administered orally it tastes horrible, but is safer... also less effective. Other dangers include the risk of infection in the injection sites, Liver failure, and sudden (paradoxically) very low blood pressure causing unconsciousness (Blackouts) and like any substance there are the risks of a severe allergic reaction. These side effects and risks are far higher when the patient is a child and that is one reason why Chelation is such a controversial area of medicine.

As a result, three better Chelators with fewer (but still significant) side effects were developed and are still widely used. One is DSMA, the second, EDTA and thirdly, DMPS—all very long sciencey names.

DMSA is best for Lead. EDTA is used for most metals, which include the "soft" metals like Calcium, Magnesium and Lithium, among others.

All three can be taken by mouth but twenty to fifty, 2-4 hour IV sessions two or three times a week is the usual method of delivery for EDTA. The patient can walk around, watch Television or read while the IV is working. DMPS is used for Mercury; it is dangerous and not licensed by the American FDA (Federal Drug Administration).

Orally, the process takes months, even years and is not as effective as by IV, really oral chelation works best as a prophylactic (prevention) action rather than a remedial one, compared with IV delivery. That said, a high daily dosage of Vitamin C (2000+milligrams (mg) per day for an adult) and some other vitamins, minerals and herbs have shown promise as natural, gentle and effective Chelators of a number of toxins and metals.

Chelation and Autism:

There are doctors and parents who believe both childhood and adult autism can be "cured" by "flushing the body" of toxic elements, especially metals and indeed there have been one or two well-reported success stories to tell from this approach. Please remember that these Chelators are powerful, unpleasant, dangerous chemicals in themselves, developed specifically for military and industrial emergency situations- and for ADULT USE. Children have died or been horribly damaged by them. To chelate a child is child abuse and endangerment of the worst type. So too is giving ANYONE another very dangerous, often fatal and very poisonous pseudo-cure, namely the poisonous sink and bathroom cleaner, Bleach (Hydrogen Peroxide) in any manner or way.

With Chelation there is no way of predicting or controlling the results. For this reason, I would never sanction its use, except when the patient, child or adult has direct blood-test or eye-witness proof of high metal/gas exposure-from whatever source. Whether the person is overtly autistic or not, should never be a part of that decision-making process. Nevertheless, as already mentioned, successes have happened. My guess is that the patients were made NLD by prior toxic exposure; perhaps gradually over time before the treatment began. In these cases, it could well help, but only in a few cases where the autism-like (NLD) symptoms were proved to be caused by poisoning.

There have not yet been sufficient high-quality clinical trials to put a figure on that "few." With any other of the causes we have discussed it is a futile and dangerous risk and I am against it. Furthermore, chelation is not a legally approved therapy for Autism in any major country which, of course, does not stop its use by greedy private or unlicensed so-called "clinics."

Author's Note: Scarily, DMPS is actually available over the counter in some countries.

Case Study 2: Is there another use for adult chelation outside of emergencies?

The answer is "Maybe": using EDTA to chelate calcium, magnesium and aluminum from the veins and arteries, gently for older people may help or prevent Parkinson's, Alzheimer's and those fatty blockages that cause strokes and heart attacks because a lot of the plaques which cause the arterial hardening (not all) and brain damage are composed partly of those elements, in combination with some fats a.k.a. Lipids and some very specific types of protein. EDTA can act like penetrating fluid, or kettle-descaler, which chemically speaking, is pretty much what it is. It can clean out the pipes, basically.

In some countries EDTA is used legally to clear blocked coronary (Heart) arteries as a cheaper, effective, and less invasive option than open-heart surgery. It is certainly not a mainstream treatment (although it is used widely across the United States, Canada and in Japan).

I am mentioning it on the basis that it works in preventing some heart attacks and dementia in the senior's age bracket which we have discussed. Once again, there is as yet insufficient clinical evidence to form a clear opinion. That said, there is enough to connect hard water with brain disease and heart attacks.

An experiment to try at home:

Take a glass, fill it with your normal drinking water, leave it 15 minutes, tip the water out and leave to dry. Check for residual scaling in the morning by holding it up to a light source, if it's cloudy—that's likely to be calcium and magnesium just from the few drops left after tipping.

Author's question: Are hardened and blocked blood vessels more common among people whose water supply is high in calcium (and/or Magnesium) than those whose water is low in it? The answer, according to a 1996 study done in Glasgow, Scotland and Washington in 2002, as well as the opinion of America's world-renowned Mayo clinic strongly indicate that a YES! I advise those in "hard water" regions to drink distilled or filtered water. An expensive filter system or jug works well but is not essential. Cheap, large filter papers bought from a chemist or general store do the same job just as effectively. Put the large cone-shaped paper inside a cheap plastic funnel; slowly pour the water through it into your normal glass and drink. Each paper can be dried, brushed, and used quite a few times for economy. Once again, the younger the person the more important this is, but any general health-risk reduction must be a good idea at every age.

Boiling water takes out a lot, but not all the impurities in it as well as killing any lurking germs in your supply and removing chlorine. There is an assumption that well, river and bottled water, whether mineral or not, is always safe. That is not necessarily true, all can contain high levels of minerals, metals and other elements, as well as bacterial or poison contamination. Fish do not climb out of the pond to use the bathroom. :) In many regions household faucet water can be the best.

****

Aspie Myth Busted: "Aspies and other Autists are deceitful and creepy because they avoid eye contact or stare at people." Well yes, we do avoid eye contact, that is one of the diagnostic signs of autism and we do tend to look at people's right shoulders, so what? It doesn't make us creepy, rude or not listening, and it isn't an indication that we're not to be trusted.

Once again with these stupid myths the complete opposite is true. Autists are known to be more trusting, trustworthy, honorable, open-minded, reliable, sincere and loyal than average, because we always lack normal social understandings. That naivety makes us far less likely to be successful con-artists, deceivers or manipulators. It also means that Autists are much more vulnerable to be taken advantage of and conned out of their money and productive talents. They are also very emotionally and therefore sexually vulnerable as well.

Secondly, one of the defining characteristics of Asperger's is an unsettlingly piercing gaze, something for which Sir Isaac Newton was noted and which some people find intimidating. That apparent "staring" thing comes partly from the fact that Autists/Aspies blink much less often than normal people and can concentrate more intently. That is not a valid excuse to discriminate against, exploit or act with hostility towards us. Again, Autists are much more likely to be the victims of crime than the perpetrators.

Autistic Fact: Autistic/AS people often have one or more of the five senses (touch, smell, hearing, sight, and taste) unusually well-developed. In my case it's hearing—I can hear dog-whistles and other higher pitches—but struggle more with the lower ends of the hearing scale.

* My hearing range is normal length, but starts and ends at abnormal levels.

Gaslighting:

Appallingly both children and adults are STILL being locked away (sometimes for LIFE) in Psychiatric units because their hyper-senses were misdiagnosed as a type of hallucination, when it isn't.

There are bad and greedy psychiatrists, paid-by-numbers out there as well. Telling a person, adult or child that they are mentally ill or incapable when they aren't is known in the ND community as **"Gaslighting."** Doing things like falsifying past events in order to manipulate and gain power over someone is an example. The "wanting-to-please/be accepted" trusting Autist personality is very vulnerable to this kind of brainwashing. Be warned; it is one of the most despicable things one person can do to another—yet professionals, family and others do it all the time, sometimes with good intentions, but more often for financial or sexual motives.

Chapter 7: The Genetic Roots of Classical Autism and Neurodiversity

There are three purposes to this chapter; initially it is an introduction to the basics of how human genetics work in general and affect autism in all its forms in particular. It then looks at the most common expressions in the subject, unravelling some obscure science terms along the way. It is not an attempt, by any means to explain fully, what is a massively complex bio-chemical field. Thirdly, it is to prepare the ground for some original thoughts and theories in the following two chapters. The first deals with why autism may transfer from x parents to their children, and yet not from y parents with a similar genetic profile. The succeeding chapter is a brand new causal theory for and explanation of at least some cases of autism/AS and NLDs-of all types developing at any stage of life as the direct result of a bio-chemical chain of events, some of which we have already examined and some we have not and is hoped be of special interest to Veterans and their families everywhere.

By means of an introduction to the practical genetics of autism, it is worth looking at the simplest inherited non-autistic condition which also very often goes hand-in-hand with autism as a co-morbidity; namely Factor-X Syndrome (FXS). William's Syndrome, as we know, is caused by multiple gene errors on just one Chromosome. Autism/AS are caused by a combination of multiple gene errors on several Chromosomes, making both very difficult to study.

FXS on the other hand is caused by just a single error on a single gene named FMR1, on the X (Female) Chromosome. The X and Y pair of Chromosomes determine our gender. A baby with two X's is female, one with an X and a Y is male. As such it is much easier to investigate than multiple gene/Chromosome conditions and by so doing scientists are able to learn much more about how genetics works in other situations, as its operating principles remain consistent throughout the whole genome, with its staggering one billion combinations of "characters."

To help understand genetics and the human genome itself, a good starting place is Matt Ridley's book, *Genome* (2000). This is widely regarded as an excellent and fun primer to the subject. He looks at various elements using each Chromosome to illustrate the chapter subject.

It starts with the nature of DNA, explaining the four basic ACGT protein building blocks of all life, (Adenine, Cytosine, Guanine and Thymine). From combinations of any three of these always e.g. AAC, every cell in us is built and placed according to its function. He then explores such diverse topics as the history of the subject: beginning with the nineteenth century monk Gregor Mendel who discovered the idea of "inheritance" by working with fruit flies through to the discovery of the purpose of DNA by Francis Crick and James Watson at Cambridge in 1953 that won both of them Nobel Prizes. He next looks at the mechanics of how it works and then on to the first successful reading of the complete human genome in December 1999. This event was in itself the inspiration behind many books, including one by the project leaders, The Sanger Institute at Cambridge University sponsored by The Wellcome Foundation.

The discovery was led by the 2002 Nobel Prize winning biologist Prof. Sir John Sulston and the Cold Spring Harbor Laboratory in New York State, USA, led by the same Prof. James Watson, the co-discoverer of DNA. Along the way, Ridley steers us through some of the specialist topics of the subject, such as how genes are named and the functions of some of the more obscure ones, the *Shank3* being a special example to which we shall return.

This shows plainly two vital things; firstly, how complex the subject is "There are one billion words {characters} in the (Human instruction book... {genome}...which makes it as long as 800 Bibles. If I read the genome out to you at the rate of one word per second, for eight hours a day, it would take a century" (Ridley,

2000). Secondly, and perhaps even more excitingly for the researcher, it illustrates how much more there is for us to learn—and how much opportunity there is for truly pioneering and world—shaking discoveries and treatments waiting for us within the subject. Imagine the designs and images you could create from a one-billion-piece, four-color Lego ™ game set.

Currently we have read the full "instruction book" of the human genome but have still to put it all in the correct order. We do not understand much about how one part affects the others and hence the overall function of the organism (human or otherwise). The genome, to some extent, resembles a quaternary machine code (a four-character code, unlike, say, the simple computer/LLM base code which is binary—zero and one).

Many analogies have been drawn to illustrate its structure. One, to highlight the complexity of the challenge facing researchers was made concerning the corn genome by Professor Patrick Schnable. He is a Baker Professor of Agronomy and director of the Center for Plant Genomics and the Center for Carbon Capturing Crops, at Iowa State University. Schnable likened it to a jigsaw puzzle.

It is a very big one and it takes immense computer power and time to assemble the final picture correctly. Due to its size, the task of scanning and compiling the entire human code has been broken down into designated genomic "territories" each of which is being sequenced and finished by different University teams (with some private companies) around the world. The findings of these teams constantly provide both the latest knowledge and the interpretations of its meaning; bearing in mind new discoveries are being made nearly every day.

Because this book is in part about the genetics that affect autism, it is mainly the teams working on those relevant chromosomes that we'll be looking at. The first is based at Stanford University in California, a pivotal member of which is Dr. Donna Spiker. In a 1999 lecture, Dr. Spiker, Clinical Director of the Stanford University Autism Research Program, speaking about the families of Fragile X Syndrome sufferers, explained "They have a risk 50-75 times greater than the general population (of Autism). These families may exhibit a genetic form of autism. That is, to pass along autism through their genes."

Alongside her perfect definition of genetic inheritance, she makes a vital point about autism, Fragile X is not an autistic condition, but in an astonishingly high sixteen percent of cases, the sufferer is severely or profoundly autistic as well. To emphasize the significance of that 16%, we are reminded that the average incidence of autism in the general population is, according to the American Society of Autism (ASA) is only that 1%. From Dr. Spiker we learn that classical autism can be inherited as a side effect or vector from other different heritable conditions and not just by a complex but by a simple specific Chromosomic recoding.

This reveals both the full scope of the issue and again fully highlights its relevance, not just for those teaching or caring for single-syndrome autistics, but for multi-syndrome ones as well and some non-autistic people like Fragile X patients. FXS children are always physically (often severely) disabled, have ADHD, elongated ears and faces, mental incapacity, reproductive deformities, very high anxiety levels (which is also true of all autistic and AS people) aggression, foot problems, shyness (like Aspies), heart problems and epilepsy-and that like Autism, boys are far more likely to inherit it than girls. We don't know why, but perhaps Prof. Baron-Cohen's theory of fetal testosterone exposure is, at least a factor behind that statistic?

The next major group to look at is the archives of the *Online Mendelian Inheritance in Man* project, named after Gregor Mendel (OMIM, 2005). These are the internet published findings of the team working at Johns Hopkins University in Maryland, spearheaded by Dr. Victor McKusick. It is a vast database of all known human genes, together with a map-like grid reference on the genome and with full clinical and experimental descriptions of what they are known to do. OMIM is a close collaborator with Medline. Medline/ PubMed is a highly popular and very reputable website covering every facet of medicine and is well worth checking out. I also reference WebMD.com

All types of Classical Autism are caused by a number of code errors on more than one gene and Chromosomes which cumulatively cause enough difference to be recognizable as autism, or, of course any other inherited trait, like eye color. To take a topical example: to confirm the discovery of the remains of King Richard III of England in February 2013 the Leicester University archaeological team responsible for the finding needed to compare the DNA of the remains with that of a known living relative. The relative who confirmed the germ line was a Canadian gentleman, Mr. Michael Ibsen, a direct descendant of Richard's eldest sister, Anne of York.

When the King's face was finally reconstructed, the resemblance, even after five centuries of generations between him and Mr. Ibsen was simply breath-taking and shows the awesome power of our genes. Our genes give us our most basic form as individuals, our "Hard wiring," our personality, our inheritance. We are largely the product of them. This tells us a lot about autism as a condition. If we can inherit features, we inherit conditions and tendencies. Nothing is in isolation. The combinations of code which makes classical autism makes the person different in other ways too, not only by "ordering" a different brain structure but by changing that of everything else. That is what makes Autism a "Whole Body Condition," because it affects not only the brain, but all other physical functions as well. This is one example gene, which forms part of that equation. AUTS4 is found at 15q11-13q (Chromosome 15) on the genome.

Author's note: I'm looking to keep these arcane names to a minimum except where they serve a strong purpose. They pinpoint the physical position of each gene within the double helix structure of our DNA, as shown in the illustration sections of this book.

That same gene also predisposes people to Glaucoma, Large Cell Lymphoma and significantly for this book, Celiac disease, among many others. The issue of "predisposition or "susceptibility" here is important. Having a certain gene does not always mean the person will have the related condition, those cases are known as "dormancy." It does mean though, as do incidences of spontaneous mutation and Epigenetic mutation that they-the "carriers" can pass it on to subsequent generations "down the germ line," who may suffer from it later.

Returning to the issue of the Shank3 gene, found on Chromosome 22-q3. This work introduces us to another team, that of Professor Thomas Bourgeron at the famous Pasteur Institute in Paris, France. Bourgeron believes autism to be a neurosynaptic condition and discovered that many autistic people and especially those with Asperger's Syndrome have a double copy of that gene's sequence. Brain imaging has proved that those people's brain synapses are structurally different from the average in the regions which deal with certain social and cognitive tasks. This makes Shank3 an excellent causal candidate for some aspects of autism. If and until larger studies can verify Prof. Bourgeron's findings, we can't be sure, as a majority of our genes are involved with, to a greater or lesser degree, the development of our brain.

Other teams working at Cambridge, Newcastle and Cardiff in the UK have noted sequence abnormalities consistent with autism on Chromosomes 2, 3, 6, 12, 15 and 20. The most likely scenario is that enough abnormalities cause autism and that the places where they occur determine the specific condition, for example, AuHD (Autism &ADHD). Dr. Fred Volkmar, Head of Child Medicine at Yale University and one of the world's leading specialists in Autism, believes that up to six major genes and as many as thirty minor ones are involved scattered across several Chromosomes with each playing a role (*Nature Genetics,* 2007). I think, from my latest genetic research that is a big underestimate, and that the gene figure will, when finally read, be above 300.

Briefly, we inherit twenty-three sets of Chromosomes from each parent, making 23 pairs. Each Chromosome contains a number of genes, a few hundred in some, a few thousand in others. All in all, a person has around 15,000 genes. All of these are known collectively as "The human Genome," and are contained in our RNA and DNA. DNA is the program (code) which, via different types of RNA- a series of chemical messengers, traffic wardens and interpreters; telling each cell what to be and where to go to assemble a complete human being, mouse, tree or whatever, like assembling a giant 3D jigsaw, as Dr. Schnable says.

Each gene and each sequence (chain) of genes does something different, or nothing, if they remain switched off, (dormant) which a lot do.

The genes that are switched on are said to be "Expressed" to make them build their assigned piece of the body at a pre-determined time during development. After all there would be no point in building a leg before the heart or brain. If at any point the code is faulty or becomes corrupted by, for example radiation, programming errors will occur and these are the genetic diseases and weaknesses which are often in the news. The same principle applies with our flat-pack parallel, if some of the pieces are wrong, or put in the wrong places; the result will be different from the picture on the box.

The genome—and this is really important to know—is active throughout the whole of life, from the moment of conception onwards and can be affected by genes being switched on or off at any time (changing the body and mind) by various factors including the toxins we have discussed and the therapies we'll look at a bit later.

Another way of thinking about the genome is to imagine a giant keyboard, each key being a gene. The tune(s) played depends on which keys are hit and when.

It is not only negative influences that can trigger conditions, so too can positive ones-the birth of a child, winning a big career promotion or gaining fame, by the same mechanism-things change, for good or bad, sometimes in profound ways.

Genetic and Autie Fact: There is even a gene that determines whether our earwax is hard or soft, it's called ABCCII discovered by scientists at Nagasaki University in Japan in 2006. Autists by observational and medical research have been shown to produce more earwax than NTs and need to have their ears checked-and flushed regularly-my recommendation is every three months. Excess or impacted earwax can cause loss of balance, which may be mis-interpreted as "clumsiness," as well as hearing difficulty, which interferes with education and general communication.

It has also long been observed by some specialists that autistics seem more likely to be borderline or actually anemic (a lack of the oxygen-carrying red blood cells in the body) causing tiredness and general malaise which may be easily misdiagnosed as "depression" or "malingering." It's another example of the Whole Body Condition. The reason is that the Autistic gut cannot properly absorb certain foods properly. Again: test and if necessary, take supplements.

Fun Fact: The common potato has 24 pairs of chromosomes.

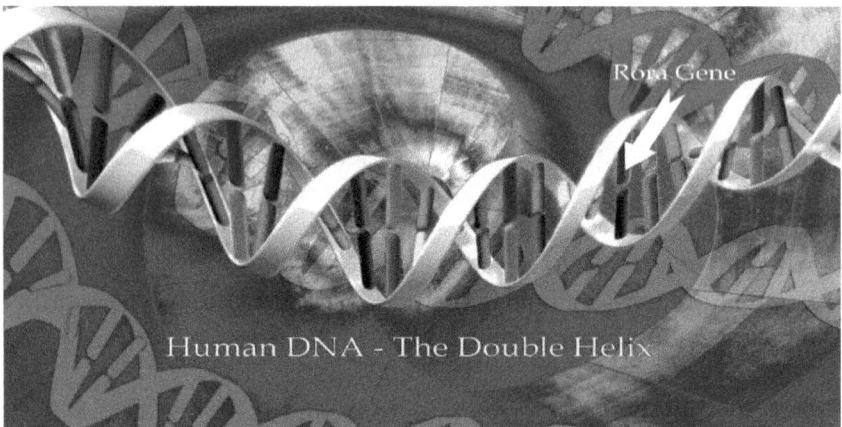

Featuring a RORA gene

Chapter 8: OCD, Electric Lights and a Cat Named Smike

Genetic expression can be influenced at any time by physical and emotional as well as toxic intervention-if the relevant genetic sequence for that change is in your individual genome already or occurs by spontaneous mutation.

Throughout the ages there have been rare but well-documented and photographed instances of people whose hair has turned white overnight after a traumatic experience, such as the death of a sibling, spouse, an accident, the loss of a long-cherished family pet, or carer, especially in Autists. The shock switches on all the genes for gray hair at once rather than over a period of years as normally happens. It happened to Shah Jehan, the builder of the Taj Mahal in Agra, India on hearing of the death of his wife, Muntez. Exactly the same applies when someone's hair drops out overnight. Cancer can be triggered by shock. All those people had the sequences disposing them to greyness, cancer or baldness, otherwise it could not have happened, they just needed "the trigger" the same is equally true of dozens of other conditions.

OCD-Obsessional Compulsive Disorder:

It can be a ritualized form of stammer, facial or other tic and Tourette's. It is, as we saw from the DSMs and ICD particularly likely to affect autistic and other Neuro-diverse groups because of the psychological trait of searching for security within fixed routines-which is helpful and healthy...up to a certain point. That point is breached when the routine rules the person's life, rather than stabilizing it.

OCD is manifested by the extreme, sometimes life disrupting expressions in the stereotyped and constant repetition of behaviors, patterns/subjects of thought, as well as to the compulsive sticking to pointless and even self-defeating routines, tasks and lifestyle choices. Doing things in a set order, being obsessive about the placement of objects on a shelf or in a room and many more, such as hoarding newspapers or cleaning dishes, adjusting pictures hundreds of times a day are common examples; in other words, actions that alienate a person from society and destroys their life.

Clearly such a person is unlikely to find employment or companionship among others. All OCD has anxiety as its root, another very autistic trait as we know. When OCD presents in someone who has already been diagnosed as autistic, doctors call it Obsessive Compulsive Personality Disorder (OCPD) to distinguish it from those exact same symptoms in non-Autists.

"The roots of compulsive behavior are always found in the experience of fear or trauma". (I. Hale).

Given the way that Autists are treated, it is obvious how we become so traumatized and why typically OCD starts so young, usually around puberty, it is clear that there is a strong link between childhood trauma and later OCD.

OCD's manifestations in non- autistic people are mainly superstitions, like wearing lucky charms, not walking under ladders, touching someone with curly hair and some of the rituals top sports players do whilst playing. A good example is how the great Russian tennis champion, Maria Sharapova carefully avoided walking on the court lines between points and games, the Spanish legend, Rafael Nadal too, has elaborate rituals on court. Cricketers' rituals make an outstanding study in OCPD.

There are two important things to note about these. Firstly, they enhance and not destroy the person's performance and focus and secondly, they are perfectly innocent and no-one else's business. There's nothing wrong with any healthy routine that works for you; these things only become an issue at the point where they make normal life hard or impossible for yourself or others. Interestingly, studies have shown that people with OCD tend to be, while socially dysfunctional, very meticulous, very good at detail, very determined and of above average intelligence-just like HFAs,

Aspies and Schizophrenics. Are there genetic links between the three? It seems increasingly likely but needs more research. Perhaps, after all they were right originally to view Asperger's as a mild form of schizophrenia. With today's rapid progress in genetics, we will soon know for sure, one way or the other.

However, severe OCDs are, with help, often beatable. I know because I had one. Let's be very honest, an OCD is a form of addiction, pure and simple. The result of performing the compulsive acts—whatever they are—is the relief of anxiety and the accompanying euphoric pleasure caused by the feeling of "being in control" of a situation or experience which has or does cause extreme fear. Doing the rituals and relieving the fear releases chemicals in the brain called endorphins—the natural "highs"/"uppers," similar to the effects of taking heroin. People who work out hard in the gym or run get that same high, for the same reason, it's very addictive and as a result very tough to beat.

Case Study 3: My compulsion was switching on and off electric light switches of any kind, mainly clandestinely at home. I would wait until my parents were asleep, and then tiptoe barefoot around the house, checking every switch and flicking them on and off up to a hundred or more times each including the outside ones; which was horrible, especially during the cold, wet, windswept English winters. This started around the age of eleven, when we moved from a single level bungalow into a two-storey house and continued into my late 20's when some people at work spotted the same behavior there.

The first few times I laughed it off, then after a couple more times realized that it was potentially a career-breaker.

Colleagues were beginning to talk about it and ask if I had a problem, or wanted to speak to a counsellor...which I didn't! I felt ashamed and angry that I had been "found out," and was afraid it would go against my career record and damage future prospects-a not uncommon thing, as I have learned from countless clients since—plus counsellors are usually expensive. The worst thing was that I had no control over it at all, because I had no idea why I was doing it, just that without it, I couldn't concentrate, eat, sleep, relax-a common problem for Autists of all types for many reasons.

I read up on the subject from some books recommended by my boss—a wonderful lady who happened to be the senior psychology lecturer—I was teaching in a college at the time... They gave me the first and most important steps to beating OCD or any other addiction-the understanding and acceptance that I had a real problem, secondly that other people had it too, and thirdly that I had a very strong motive to overcome it.

So I thought and read the books about it-over months and at the same time tried to fight—which didn't work—it just made me very irritable, stressed and shaky although I did force myself to semi-stop at work, but increased the behavior outside—so even more people thought I was "strange" (ha-ha). Then one day during a coffee break, I suddenly remembered the key to it all in a lengthy and vivid flashback. I was asleep at home aged about five or six and only recently back from hospital after having my appendix out—which in itself was traumatic.

I woke up to foul-smelling smoke and flames and sparks coming from the bedroom light switch—which was too high for me to reach. I ran into my parents' bedroom and woke them up—still in pain from the recently-removed stitches... my Dad came in, opened the window, switched the house electricity off, put the fire out, and then tied off and wrapped insulation tape round all the wiring as I knelt on the end of the bed and watched. In the morning, he showed me what had happened. It was a cheap brown plastic switch fitment, with frayed, cotton-coated old-fashioned brown wiring, that had shorted out and caught fire, setting the switch alight, which then melted the plastic. The house was only seven years old but had been poorly built by a drunk sub-standard builder.

When our family moved into a two-storey house my subconscious must have recalled the event and thought, "suppose it happens again here, downstairs in the night and we are all asleep upstairs, we we'll all burn to death." At that moment I was released from it. I had seen the face of fear and realized that in modern, properly inspected buildings, at home or at work, it just wasn't going to happen again. I have not had such behavior or anything similar since. That sense, during the coffee break of discarding the shackles of two decades, left me crying and shaking for days, on and off.

I was lucky that the combination of reading, self-analysis and the support of professional colleagues created that coffee-break epiphany. For people without such support, counselling with a professional, specialist analyst can be equally useful. I am, from professional experience extremely cynical regarding the use of group therapy, CBT (Cognitive Behavioral Therapy), and the other cost-cutting, half-baked forms of "social care therapy."

I strongly oppose any type of "conversion" behavioral therapies, especially Autism Behavioral Therapy (ABT), for adults and, especially children. They all aim to teach or force new ways of thinking and acting on the child to fit in better with what society wants, not what they need. They all go against our individual "Hard-wiring," many involve beating, electrocuting and slapping the child to "behave", as the so-called therapist wants, causing life-long psychological havoc. **I am against ANY form of force or coercion, whether it's called "therapy" or not, especially when it is abuse-based.** We are who we are as individuals and have the right to develop naturally in our own time and way.

If proper one-on-one counselling is not possible or wanted then a skilled, certified hypnotist who by "regressing" the mind down the memory of the years may find the event(s) which lie at the core of a person's psychic fear and, by exposing it, make it fight-able. The process is called "running the trauma."

I have seen and many done private and live, successful demonstrations of its positive effectiveness.

There are also prescribed Psycho-active (those which affect the brain) medications which can alleviate the symptoms of OCD. The most likely to be prescribed is a Selective Serotonin Re-uptake inhibitor (SSRI) such as Celexa, Paxil or Prozac. These drugs act to both stabilize mood swings and as antidepressants. They are "chill-out" pills and can be very beneficial and life-empowering for some people, yet non-effective or damaging to others. The drugs act by fooling the brain into thinking it has more Serotonin (the happy chemical) than it does, making it act that way. The prevailing theory (and it is only a theory, not a proven fact) is that low Serotonin levels are the cause of clinical depression, which can trigger anxiety and hence OCD.

However, like most drugs they have side-effects, including loss of self-motivation, self-esteem, lethargy, nausea, a well-documented increased risk of suicide, rashes (sometimes) and loss of sex drive (Libido). On top of those, they tend to be addictive and can cause long term liver damage. I feel, as with Ritalin for ADD that they should only be used as a treatment of last resort in the most challenging of cases and under the strictest supervision, for the shortest possible period of time.

* Interestingly, two large 2025 published studies indicate that SSRIs taken young clearly decrease the risk of dementia in later life.

The second preferred type of drug to relieve all types of anxiety (Antiaxiolytics) are the Benzodiazepines; the most popular and best of which, in my opinion is Xanax, made by the Pfizer Company of Brooklyn, New York. Appropriate instances for this drug treatment are people who find they are either unwilling or unable to talk about their experiences because it makes them feel worse by constantly re-stimulating the original trauma to unbearable levels. It is a normal and not terribly uncommon situation; especially as such people usually have PTSD as a co-morbidity. For some, hypnosis may not be possible or do more harm than good by re-stimulation or if someone's memory has become so deeply buried in the subconscious that it is unreachable.

Case Study 4: Smike was a tiny, black, rain-soaked, starving cat who my parents found in a gutter one evening and adopted, years before I was born.

They wrapped him in a small towel, fed him and put him in a little basket near the fireside. Over time, with love and care he got better and bigger and they called him "Smike" after the poor boy who Nicholas befriends in Charles Dickens' novel, *Nicholas Nickleby.*

For a year or two afterwards, every time they did cleaning, moved furniture and sometimes outside, they found little cached hoards of food that Smike had hidden away from the memories of his hard times and treatment. Later on, fully settled and content, that stopped, showing how compulsive, anxiety-driven repetitive behavior can be overcome by love, kindness, patience and trust, no matter how deep or how early the original trauma. We can all learn from that. Smike lived happily until the age of fifteen and a half. Hope is strong, hope is real.

Chapter 9: PTSD and Autism, is There a Link?

Post-Traumatic Stress Disorder-sometimes referred to as "shell shock" "survivor's guilt" or "battle fatigue," among other things. It can be caused by a single physical or emotional event such as 9/11, a violent assault, a motor accident or a series of events over a long period of time. Loss of, or separation from a loved one, bullying and abuse are the three most common sources in childhood, as we'll see later.

Horror, including being abandoned as a child, any kind of impossible family circumstances-like caring for and watching a loved one decline and die- that can include a loved animal companion, are also common causes.

When the cause is cumulative, the result is a gradual erosion of emotional reserves-some psychologists call it Complex-PTSD or "Burnout."

In either situation, both the ICD and DSM are more-or-less in agreement on its telltale signs and symptoms. It can be likened to a battery being drained, leaving the person, unresponsive, numbed out, and lacking "spark" or any enjoyment of life.

There is nothing new about PTSD; the modern definitions below have been recorded down the ages by contemporaries, historians, observers and ordinary citizens in people who have survived earthquakes, volcanoes, floods and other natural disasters, as well as soldiers, airmen and sailors returned from war. Hannibal's chroniclers record it and Hannibal sent affected soldiers home to recover.

PTSD is normal; it is not a sign of weakness. *"Weakness is when a person denies it and does not seek help. The truly strong confront it and do something-that is courage, the acceptance of one's humanity"* (**I. Hale**).

The DSM criteria for PTSD are:

A. The person has been exposed to a traumatic event(s) in which both of the following have been present:

(1) The person experienced, witnessed, or was confronted with an event or events that involved actual or threatened death or serious injury, or a threat to the physical integrity of the self or others

(2) The person's response involved intense fear, helplessness, or horror. Note: in children, this may be expressed instead by disorganized or agitated behavior. *Author's note*: perhaps, in many cases mistaken for ADHD???

B. The traumatic event is persistently re-experienced in one (or more) of the following ways:

(1) Recurrent and intrusive distressing recollections of the event, including images, thoughts, or perceptions. Note: in young children, repetitive play may occur in which themes or aspects of the trauma are expressed:

Author's note: another strongly Autistic trait, the evidence mounts.

(2) Recurrent distressing dreams of the event. Note: In children, there may be sleep-walking and/or frightening dreams without recognizable content sometimes called "Night terrors," which may also be caused by an undiagnosed physical illness. Fast, professional help is vital in either situation.

(3) Acting or feeling as if the traumatic event was recurring (including a sense of reliving the experience, illusions, hallucinations, and dissociative flashback episodes, including those that occur upon awakening or when intoxicated). Note: in young children, trauma-specific re-enactment may occur.

(They re-live the experience) – I. Hale.

(4) Intense psychological distress at exposure to internal or external cues that symbolize or resemble an aspect of the traumatic event.

(5) Physiological reactivity on exposure to internal or external cues that symbolize or resemble an aspect of the traumatic event.

C. Persistent avoidance of stimuli associated with the trauma and numbing of general responsiveness (not present before the trauma), as indicated by three (or more) of the following:

(1) Efforts to avoid thoughts, feelings, or conversations associated with the trauma.

(2) Inability to recall an important aspect of the trauma.

(3) Efforts to avoid activities, places, or people that arouse recollections of the trauma.

(4) Markedly diminished interest or participation in significant activities. Feelings of detachment or estrangement from others.

(5) Restricted range of affect (e.g., unable to have loving feelings, some say that of Autists).

(6) A sense of a foreshortened future (e.g., does not expect to have a career, marriage, children, or a normal life span).

D. Persistent symptoms of increased arousal (not present before the trauma), as indicated by two (or more) of the following:

(1) Difficulty falling or staying asleep.

(2) Irritability or outbursts of anger.

(3) Difficulty concentrating.

(4) hyper-vigilance (always "keyed up and can't relax or let their guard down" – *author's note*).

(5) Exaggerated "startle response."

That "startle response" is the prime indicator of the condition. You get the patient to chat, relax, have a cup of tea and ask an assistant, unnoticed, to tap them lightly on the shoulder, or make a sharp noise. If the person "jumps" obviously, PTSD is basically confirmed.

E. Duration of the disturbance (symptoms in Criteria B, C, and D) is more than one month.

F. The disturbance causes clinically significant distress or impairment in social, occupational, or other important areas of functioning.

The ICD (v 10) section F43, says almost exactly the same things; there is no need to repeat them. The important thing to bear in mind is that the patient was perfectly healthy before the event(s) which triggered their condition. There are two answers to the question of whether there is a link between PTSD and Autism, one of them is a near definite "yes" and the second, in this author's experience is also clearly "yes."

Firstly, a team at Boston University supported by the American V.A. (Veteran's Affairs, who, despite underfunding, attempt to care for ex-service people) led by Dr. Mark Miller, a specialist clinical psychologist. Dr. Miller studied the genomes of hundreds of traumatized Veterans and other volunteers before publishing a preliminary report in *"VA Research Currents"* online magazine in August, 2012. He found a statistically significant number of his PTSD patients compared with the healthy volunteers carried one particular sub-type of the RORA gene, which expresses in the brain and affects our emotional states and responses, among other things. This and many other sub-types of RORA figure prominently in the genomes of Autists, especially HFAs, and

Aspies, making the RORA genes among prime candidates for being part of the "autism genome," as predicted by Drs Volkmar and Bourgeron and further supported by the research of Dr. Christopher Badcock, of the London School of Economics (LSE) one of Britain's top Universities, as he explained in his book, *"The imprinted Brain"* (2009)

This gives us a firmer indication as to why some people are more likely than others to suffer PTSD in any given situation, or pass on autism to their children. Also, it may explain why two people may suffer the same traumatic experience with one going on to develop PTSD while the other does not. It could explain why autistic people are more likely than NTs to experience PTSD and why many of the PTSD symptoms- the marked increased risk of suicide being one- match those of Autism/AS and ADHD, notably being emotionally "closed in"-unresponsive. These conditions appear to derive from the same or similar specific genetic sequences.

From this I believe derives the second "yes," linking PTSD to Autism- that traumatic experiences can cause autism/NLD as well as its other noted effects to develop at any age. It does it by activating previously dormant genes already in certain people to suddenly express, causing autism to present. This process could be caused by a variety of stressors; Toxins or life-changing experiences whether they are negative like trauma, or positive, like a huge lottery win.

These same changes can also occur due to a second genetic process at work, namely Epigenetics. Epigenetic change is not the changing of the DNA sequencing itself from within. It is changes and mutations caused by external factor(s). Things like toxic exposures, excess sun tanning, excess fat etc. As with Autism, these affect the genome and therefore physical and mental health, via gene "expression." Those changes may or may not be passed on down to future generations. PTSD can be caused by this process-and who knows, maybe others too.

The influential nineteenth century German philosopher Freidrich Nietzsche wrote "that which doesn't kill us, makes us stronger." He should have added... "or gives us PTSD, Depression and/or Autism and perhaps our children, grandchildren and great-grandchildren as well." Again, we must stress the universal lesson that genetics teaches us: that there is no blame, no weakness, no stigma and no shame in any of these things, just a combination of biophysics, a suitable "trigger" and "susceptibility."

"One thing affects everything, big and small, good and bad. From this understanding emerges tolerance and compassion, from these we should kindle the fires of hope and progress" (I. Hale).

Further evidence for this process comes from the fact that stress has well proven links to cancer; heart attacks and to triggering Shingles in people who carry the Chickenpox virus, all by damaging their immune systems. These are all purely physical manifestations. I submit that by the same argument, trauma can trigger autism, because it has clear physical causes lying deep within the human brain. By that self-same mechanism PTSD also has clear external physical causes and manifestations within the brain, including, as has already been medically established.

Take TBIs: Professor Tian Xu, a geneticist at Yale University said: "A lot of different conditions can trigger stress signaling–physical stress, emotional stress, infections, inflammation–all these things." Reducing stress or avoiding stress conditions is always good advice.

The most convincing evidence, proving that in children at least, mental and/or emotional abuse, rejection or neglect alone actually physically changes the structure of their DNA and brain to produce PTSD-like effects was conducted by the McMaster University of Ontario in Canada and was revealed by its co-author, the notable psychiatrist Dr. Harriet MacMillan in the July 30 edition of the *US News & World Report*, 2012. She wrote "The main message for child health clinicians and people working with children is that psychological maltreatment is just as harmful as other types of maltreatment." She continued...

"We know that exposure to other types of maltreatment like physical and sexual abuse can be associated with a broad range of types of impairment in physical and mental health and cognitive and social development. Similarly, we see these types of impairments associated with psychological maltreatment. The same is true of emotional abuse or the with-holding of unconditional love and of course bullying, all these affect the body as well as the mind." It is not unreasonable to suggest that lack of parental attention, too much video-gaming as well as the above could produce autistic-like behaviors, but not true, classical autism, again adding to the "epidemic" mistake.

****

A word on Shutdowns:

Finally, we noted that PTSD produces emotional numbness/deadness and lack of self-care. Autism "Shutdowns" show very similar signs. They happen in response to sensory or emotional overload and cause the person to freeze, crippled by an overwhelming but nameless anxiety, becoming physically, mentally and emotionally paralyzed for varying periods of time: minutes, hours, weeks and so on. It feels as if you're being slowly squeezed into a tight, dark muddy cave. It's a terrifying experience (I've had a number) of total powerlessness, of being trapped by your own inability to change or do anything. You need support-family, friends, and a personal advocate.

This is NOT the same as clinical depression, or worry, although it and a number of other things can trigger it. As a result, psychiatrists often make a wrong assumption and the person is forced into, inappropriate, unnecessary or downright dangerous drugs and other treatments.

Chapter 10: The Left-handed Connection

It has long been known that left-handed people are more likely to be Dyslexic than their right-handed counterparts. Left-handedness, is like classical autism genetically inherited, so in left-handed families with Dyslexia in the genes the probability of any family member being Dyslexic and left-handed is much higher than average.

Around 10% of the world's population are left-handed (*The Week*, April 27, 2012) they are more likely to be schizophrenic than the general population, but also more likely to have genius-level IQ s and/or be more artistic than right-handers. Examples include Albert Einstein, Michelangelo, Leonardo Da Vinci, Bill Gates, Sir Isaac Newton, Benjamin Franklin, and Aristotle. Guitarist and electronics inventor Jimi Hendrix, boxer Marvin Hagler, Thomas Jefferson, H G Wells, Alexander the Great, Marie Curie, Martina Navratilova, Mahatma Gandhi, Angelina Jolie, Thomas Jefferson (to whom I am blood related) and Charles Darwin.

Left-handedness is slightly less common in women than men. Lefties are more prone to addictions-principally alcohol. Jack the Ripper was left-handed, as was The Boston Strangler and the American gangster, John Dillinger.

Left-handedness also runs strongly through the British Royal Family, Queen Victoria, King George VI, The Queen Mother, Queen Elizabeth II, Prince Charles and his son Prince William were/are all left-handers.

To illustrate the lefty/Autist connection: A 1983 study by Prof. Lars C Gillberg, a leading child psychiatrist from the University of Gothenburg in Sweden, found among Autist/AS children and in comparison, with a peer group of non-autistic ones, he found 15% of left-handedness among non-autistics. But of the Autists a staggeringly high 37% were left-handed/ambidextrous, that is, being able to use both hands equally well, with neither dominant.

Similar results have been broadly replicated since by other teams, indicating in the clearest possible way that there is a firm genetic link between left-handedness and autism. Why should this be?

My pathology research has suggested one possible reason at least. The brain is actually two brains, the left and right hemispheres which are connected by a thick tissue/nerve bridge, the Corpus Callosum. In right-handed people, the left side of the brain is dominant, in lefties, the right dominates.

In cases of autism in general and AS in particular, where the structure of the left side of the brain is more commonly different from standard, or in N(S)LDs brains, left-handedness would make sense. In my case, I throw right and catch left, play cricket right, but table tennis and badminton left, Pool-both ways. Nirvana's founder and guitarist, Kurt Cobain, played left, but wrote (usually) right as does the Spanish tennis star, Rafael Nadal. Exactly the same applies to hearing and sight as to football. Auties/AS also tend to be left ear, eye and foot dominant, as compared with NTs.

We must conclude that there is a connection between dyslexia, Autism and the left-handedness. This again brings us back to the tricky debate about whether Dyslexia (and for that matter, Dyscalculia) are members of the Autism or NLD families. It seems they can be either, as not all dyslexics are autistic by any means, but quite a few autistics/AS are dyslexic. The question has as yet no definitive answer. It works on a person-by-person basis, and is one of the many contradictions in the study of Autism which science has yet to resolve and from which this book deliberately does not shrink from recognizing and reflecting.

Author's note: Please, never, **ever** try to "turn" a naturally left-handed child to conform with right-handed society, no matter how good the intention. Doing so will cause neurological confusion resulting in many potential disorders including poor co-ordination, anxiety, OCD, and sometimes self-destructive habits, depression, dyslexia and lack of muscle memory. These conditions tend to get worse as the child approaches adulthood and continue doing so throughout life, to a point where very serious mental illnesses may develop.

The correct thing to do is to encourage and re-assure the child about left-handedness and make sure that the school and staff have the materials and knowledge that are needed. If they don't, make a fuss and make/buy/adapt as much equipment at home as possible.
For example, something as simple as whittling down hexagonal pencils or crayons to being duel-sided for easier grip. Cricket bat bases are also very easy to chamfer down to left-leaning, right-hand guitars can be converted fairly easily, as can a computer mouse, there are some good instruction videos on the net.

Chapter 11: Boys and Girls

Hemophilia is sometimes known as "the bleeding disease" because the sufferer lacks the chemical (Fibrin) that makes blood clot. In the past before modern medicine, it was life-threatening, as the slightest cut, knock or bruise to the body or head could result in death. It was also nicknamed "The Royal disease"—Queen Victoria was a carrier, and her daughters spread it into almost every Royal House of Europe, most notably Portugal and Russia. The Russian Empress, Alexandra, wife of Tsar Nicholas II was a carrier and their heir, Alexis was a severe hemophiliac. The only person who seemed able to treat him and who saved his life many times was the notorious monk, Gregori Rasputin.

As a result, his influence at court grew and grew leading to jealousy from the nobility he had supplanted and horror from the Russian people because of his reportedly debauched lifestyle and rumors of an affair with Alexandra. Rasputin was murdered by a band of nobles in 1916. A year later the people rebelled in the Russian Revolution which first removed and then executed the Tsar and his whole family. It's one of those interesting historical "what ifs." If Alexis had not been a hemophiliac, there would have been no Rasputin at court and perhaps no revolution?

Hemophilia is purely a genetic condition affecting only males, because its genetic code is carried on the female X chromosome. Such single-gender conditions are unusual and called "Autosomal Dominant." For most conditions the child has to inherit a copy of the damaged gene from each parent-those are "autosomal Recessive" cases. We have seen earlier that there are genetic conditions which affect only females and others which affect the genders unequally, that is, have a strong gender bias, Autism and AS are two. This has been confirmed by the researchers Dr. Tony Attwood and Prof. Gillberg among many. The suggested ratio for Autism is just above 4.2:1 (Male) other studies have varied that figure to some extent. However, the central point that autism and

AS are far more common in males than females remains clear. The question is, why?

My thought is that AS and Autism are caused primarily from among the 200+ genes on the male Y chromosome, 72 of which are the vital base protein coders (NIH, 2013). The X and Y chromosomes are about far more than just gender determination. If that is correct it would add weight to Baron-Cohen's FT theory and my theory that Autism and particularly AS are mainly transmitted through the father's germ line by the same mechanism as blood type, and why Autism/AS is more prevalent in boys than girls. What is also clear is that when females have AS they have it on average, far more severely than males. The same is true of dyslexia, again indicating that some forms, at least of dyslexia are certainly autistic in origin, while others are not.

As diagnosis has improved, as it has since the early 1990's one might have expected to see that ratio drop for a number of reasons. In many societies female education was-and in some, still is-regarded as unimportant and girls had little or no schooling and hence little chance of being diagnosed, as the male was expected to be the breadwinner. Secondly, some symptoms of AS, in particular the avoidance of eye contact would be regarded as "proper, modest, even desirable female behavior" in some cultures, as would the quiet, home and peace-loving nature of Autists and Aspies and again go undetected. Additionally, girls are less physically aggressive and open about expressing their emotions and are, compared with boys, less likely to attract the kind of attention that would lead to a psychiatric assessment.

Basically, girls have the same symptoms as boys, but present them very differently to the outside world; far too few doctors know that.

Girls tend to mask their separation from the perceived "normal" much more effectively than boys, try harder to conform and bottle up the resulting feelings of alienation from others for decades, even for life. Doing this can result in secretive but unhealthy coping behaviors; substance abuse, cutting and bulimia being three. That masking is another reason girls are frequently overlooked by psychologists, schools and family as Autistic or AS. Even when they do get assessed, it is all too often put down to "hysteria" or "hormones" and then ignored, when if it were a boy, the same symptoms would be instantly recognized as an autistic meltdown and supported.

To make the situation worse, diagnosis, as we've seen, comes via Evidence Based Medicine.

With the overwhelming number of men with Autism (regardless of the true ratio) compared with women, most of the existing evidence comes, naturally from male studies—that would be fine if males and females presented their symptoms the same. The trouble is they don't. Women present their symptoms and experiences and deal with them differently, as we've seen.

There's more: Take Asperger's: it is not uncommon for women with AS to be misdiagnosed with schizophrenia, because, as we've agreed, although very few have it, those who do present more severely than most male Aspies and severe AS looks a lot like schizophrenia, leading to these women being mis-medicated, mistreated and even institutionalized-for life. Yet another problem is that because of the rarity of AS in women-diagnosticians don't think to look for it, they don't ask the right questions: family history, dyslexia etc. so invariably come up with no or the wrong answer.

A further issue which needs correcting is late diagnosis-where the person is not diagnosed until far into adulthood. Mostly that applies to women, many of whom go through life unrecognized. It happens to men, but far less often, again the primary reason being because it is expected more and therefore looked for by doctors and psychologists. An example-and please feel free to disagree, this is a purely personal opinion: I think Marilyn Monroe was an undiagnosed Autist, whose mis-medication and maltreatment caused so many of the problems throughout her life.

The fact is that the male and female brains are very different, especially when processing social or emotional input. They actually use different parts of the brain to process those tasks—and as Autism/AS are essentially about social and emotional processing and women mask their symptoms so well, it does make diagnosis harder. It is up to the institutions, media and professionals as well as society at large to modify its behaviors, not ND women and girls.

The answer is for the professions to ask more questions and be more welcoming and inclusive of women. They must learn, listen and train better by bringing in and listening to the experiences of more ND women and girls, then, hopefully the diagnostic accuracy will improve. The sooner we all start doing this, the better. It has already begun in some parts of Europe, Romania, Sweden and Holland among them.

One further factor to bear in mind is that in many cultures parents were/are far less likely to send their daughters to psychiatrists for fear of stigmatizing the family with "mental illness" and reducing the chances of advantageous marriages for other siblings. Yet, as these attitudes have begun to change over more parts of the world and diagnosis become more available and accurate for girls that original male/female ratio gap has so far not changed.

We need more resources, more high-quality research and more oversight on our methods until we find a single, consistent ratio figure. Then and only then will we at least know that girls and boys are receiving the same standard of care.

Chapter 12: The Importance of Early Detection

Dr. Phillip Kendall of the Temple University in Philadelphia wrote in 2001... "Without {early} treatment the prognosis for persons with autistic disorders is not guarded.....nor do they develop the ability to interact socially in ways that are considered normal." This clearly applies to the classroom situation too. His point is further reinforced in context by Simon Franke "...it is increasingly important to develop more effective early teaching interventions...and (popular) strategies" (*In Touch*, 2007 King's College London Journal- pp12-14).

To succeed fully for each individual, diagnosis must be early, and the study of genetics can help achieve this goal. Toward this end, the teacher and scientist should work hand-in-hand. The design of this book deliberately mirrors the structure of that vital partnership in order to highlight it. Kate Wall in her brilliant *2004 Autism and Early Years Practice* asserts, "The importance of practitioner {Teacher} awareness and understanding of Autistic Spectrum Disorders is once again highlighted as a fundamental element of effective assessment and provision" That statement was an inspiration for this book's attempt to aid both awareness and diagnostics. On the subject of early recognition, she adds, "Any delays in the diagnostic process and subsequent provision will magnify the already existing problems..." There are many other examples available. Parents need to know as quickly as possible to research then choose the most appropriate school or program for their child. That may entail a house move and/or a career or role change for someone in the family. Schools need to know in plenty of time so they can plan for the child's admission and education schedule.

Social services need to know about autistic children and adults as soon as possible to be able to maximize the help available, as does the ASA in America along with similar organizations elsewhere in the world, like ASPECT (Autism Spectrum Australia) and ASAN

(Autism Self-Advocacy Network). Families need to know as early as possible, so that they too can plan and learn well in advance, as with any child. Even with genetic testing, which can only provide a statistical likelihood, formal diagnosis is very difficult before the age of two.

****

The ideal education platform for any student of whatever age, ability or gender, whether they are autistic or NT is low-ratio, student-centered learning. That is, a pupil-teacher ratio of no more than six to one and the emphasis should not be to pigeon- hole pupils into subjects or grades, but to expose them to the widest possible educational opportunities to discover their strengths and then build on those. Everyone has a thing or things they do best, this should be nurtured and time not wasted on pushing students to achieve minimum grades in things they hate. The result of this is the pernicious, State-imposed philosophy of a broad levelling down of education standards, creates bored, angry, frustrated students whose talents are ignored and who will react negatively to the experience. Increased truancy rates will be one of the many results together with the appearance of more ADD/ADHD-like behaviors' in classrooms-disruption because of boredom. The result of such a policy will be that education will be disdained, good teachers will leave and mediocrity, de-skilling, "dumbing down" and social failure will accelerate to the point of collapse.

Michelangelo said of his sculptures that his secret was to "see" the already perfect, realized work within the raw block of marble and then, with his chisel, reveal that image to the world. That's how education should work; to reveal the inner talents and that is why my argument for Personal Learning/Employment plans is so important for both the individual and society as a whole. The idea that one curriculum or style fits all pupils is nonsense. We are all individuals and should be treated as such. If reputable online or home-schooling works best for a pupil-great, the tradition of the "Sausage-factory school environment should not be considered in any way sacrosanct, nor acceptable.

That strange, eccentric child/employee, usually sitting alone in a corner, perhaps trying to attract attention might just be another Leonardo or Bill Gates and until governments, psychologists and teachers take that on board, education and social systems will fail to maximize potential-don't blame it on the child. It is probably so why many talented students drop out of school at various ages and why a lot of Aspies and HFAs become self-taught (Autodidacts).

To return to Special Education Needs… it tends to focus all its resources on people with learning difficulties. Let us not forget, as is frequently the case, those at the other end of the spectrum. The highly gifted or genius children, are just as much Special Needs as their less gifted peers. In mainstream education they are often bored, can be disruptive, bullied and their talents stifled by the imposed rigid "curriculum" system. This can be and is often mistaken for ADD/ADHD. For Aspies this exaggerates their natural tendency to leave tasks/projects uncompleted-they got bored or distracted by something else. Gentle, constant guidance can overcome this trait and foster good habits. A question worth asking of any school is "Have the teachers achieved certified skill levels in "active listening"? It is an important indicator to school quality.

If the answer is "yes" it's indicative of a good school, if not, avoid it. "Active listening" is a skill every teacher should have and is especially important in SEN staff. "Active listening" is the ability to understand what is being communicated, not only by mouth but by NVC to the extent of being able to give questioning feedback, explanation and reassurance. That shows the teacher really has grasped the full input and meaning from the pupil and not just nodded through the motions of pretending to seem empathic and interested. It's the hallmark of a really good teacher, that desire to go the extra mile for his/her pupils.

Gifted is, by definition, not "normal." I urge parents to have their child's IQ assessed as early as possible at ages 2, 5, 7, 12 and 15+, as some develop their gifts earlier or later than others. The same necessary pre-planning applies equally to these children, their carers, and in later life as adults, because for self and group advocacy it is an absolute imperative. The alternative for the majority is to be ignored or marginalized throughout their lives.

These same criteria apply to all branches of any social or community services available. The earlier they know a child's needs, the better prepared they can be. This must include the local Doctor, the police, who through lack of training and experience can sometimes be grossly abusive and/or oblivious towards Autists. They often misinterpret the unresponsiveness as guilt or defiance, when they simply do not understand the situation. Autistic people are therefore more likely than average to be involved in truancy, petty crime, parking offenses, graffitiing, and the general thing of not understanding the accepted "Social boundaries" of behavior. Their trusting natures make them the perfect patsies and victims if they get into the wrong circle of people, a fact that a lot of law enforcement, social and judicial systems either don't appreciate or simply don't consider.

The huge number of autistic people who have been fooled or bullied into confessing crimes they did not commit is shocking. To use just two cases from England to illustrate the situation. Firstly that of Barry George, freed after eight years in prison -for the murder of TV presenter, Jill Dando, a crime he did not commit- having been falsely convicted because he was an easy target for a police force under media pressure to get someone quickly, the victim being a high-profile and popular public figure. Regrettably he is not the only one.

Another is Gary McKinnon, the Scotsman who is both profoundly Asperger's and a computer wizard, who accidentally accessed the wrong US government computer files while searching for information on free energy, flying saucers and "little green men from Mars." For this—and it must be stressed he did no harm—he was arrested by the UK police in 2002 and then indicted by a Grand Jury in America then spent years under arrest trying to avoid that government's attempts to extradite him to America where he faced 70 years in jail. One wonders what they wanted to hide.

In October 2012, then British Home Secretary Theresa May (later, Prime Minister) blocked the extradition after advice from top Psychologists revealed that as an Aspie, McKinnon was highly likely to commit suicide if he was sent to America. He was not malicious; he hurt no one but was simply a man unable to grasp the political and judicial implications of his admittedly illegal actions. Would someone with a physical disability, such as failing vision who continued to drive (safely) after being advised by a doctor not to, have been treated so harshly? McKinnon has now had all charges against him dropped and works for British security.

Author's tip: Every Au person/family should seek out an attorney/Free drop-in with a specialist in handling cases involving ND clients. (I. Hale)

Autist and Aspie fact: Dr. Venkatesan (of whom much more later) has understood and campaigned about something which few others have even considered or understood. Children and adults with Autism, unlike those with, for example Cerebral Palsy are not necessarily any less disabled; it's only that the disability is not immediately obvious to the outside world. It is a "hidden disability" and people either ignore it or fail to see it. They often feel free to mock, discriminate or bully such people at will. It is as disgusting a behavior to disrespect a person with a learning disability or Autism as it would be to treat a polio victim or amputee that way.

To return to genetic testing: those on Chromosome 6 being an example, have become more widespread due to an improvement in both scientific equipment and techniques combined with an increased understanding of the cause-and-effect relationship between certain sequences and Autistic conditions. These are getting closer to the point of being available as part of regular pre-birth screening in the same way as Down's syndrome or Cerebral Palsy screens are routinely conducted today in many countries.

There are other protein-marker based tests for fetal autism being developed as this book is being written. Of course, pre-natal screening raises many moral, religious and ethical questions which are fully acknowledged, but outside the scope of this book.

Dyslexia Fact: Dyslexia affects males and females in exactly the same ratio as autism does, yet again adding more evidence towards Dyslexia being, at least in many instances part of the Autism Family, rather than wholly the NLD one.

However, I reserve some considerable doubt about that Dyslexia figure in isolation. Although Chromosome 6 has been positively identified as the carrier of a specific Dyslexic gene, experience suggests that is an incomplete picture for, as Professor Robert Plomin of King's College, London has proved—it also harbors, and not by coincidence, some of the "high intelligence, genius genes." There can, however, be no doubt that Chromosome 6 pre-disposes the male to Dyslexia should any of the "triggers" express it.

Dyslexia Tip: There are now a great many electronic aids available to help dyslexics from voice-controlled typing, to auto-text and grammar correction Apps and others, all of which are available on mobile devices as well as desk and laptop computers, they are being improved all the time. Another aid which about a third of dyslexics find helpful (including the author) are Irlen Sheets and glasses. These are A4 size colored plastic sheets which you place over a text, image or spreadsheet (it works for Dyscalculia, too) and they really can clarify it, although why is not entirely clear. They are cheap and come in a huge variety of colors; you pick the color that best helps your dyslexia and can even have prescription glasses and car windshields made with the color and…magic. :)

The conclusion to this chapter has to be to again restate the importance of early diagnosis to afford the time to prepare the correct type and amount of any interventions required to give the child or adult the best chance of maximizing both their lifetime potential and personal happiness.

There may indeed not always be a need for intervention in every case. What every case does, without exception, is both implore and demand acceptance and understanding from family, authorities and society at large. Early diagnosis gives the time to ensure that the conditions for the autistic person are optimized for all involved at all stages of their lives, including the much overlooked, elderly care.

In the next chapter we'll examine two very different psychological interpretations of the mindset of an Autist, following that, the final section of the book will look at a number of practical and sometimes very simple methods, both mainstream and from personal experience to both further explain and enrich the world of autism. To be frank, that world is seldom easy, but with some patience, knowledge, practice, imagination and determination, it can be made a lot easier to navigate than it was only a very few years ago.

That section will take a look at the future and the almost miraculous nature of the prospects which are beginning to bloom for Autists and their carers from the fields of science, psychology and education.

Autist Tip: Adult Employment: Statistically no doubt because of their weak interpersonal skills and spirit of independence—of wanting to do things "their way"—Autists often become successful by being either completely self-employed or freelance contractors who pick and choose their assignments. In the main we are not team players. Another Autistic trait, odd sleeping patterns, preferring or naturally having to sleep during the day has been turned successfully to advantage by some Autists, including Charles Darwin. But it also has another side, which again society doesn't care about. We are forced into unnatural conformity that makes school, hospitals and other rigid institutions a nightmare for us and is another reason why suicide rates are so high and follow the age group patterns they do. Among ASDs in "care homes" or prison, the rate is 67 times higher than the average. This is totally unacceptable.

Many Autists now choose unusual but regular patterns of work, night work included, but also stepped-contract work, say; 21 days straight on, 21 days off, repeating. It is easier to find as fewer people want to do them, they pay far better and there is a wider choice of work. Commuting is quicker or less frequent. A friend who is an ambulance driver is an Autist and another who is in security chose their work very carefully with their strengths and moral commitment in the forefront of their minds.

Chapter 13: Two Views on Asperger's

To return to the work of Prof. Baron-Cohen and his colleagues at the Autism Research Centre at Cambridge University on Asperger's. They conduct a number of online and face-to-face tests, interviews and surveys from a broad group of volunteers, Aspie or not and regardless of age, education, employment and gender. These increase their knowledge and understanding of the Aspie consciousness and mind in comparison with the population at large. One such test involves around 30 pictures of people's faces, some are full neck-up images, others just from brow to nose, emphasizing the expression of the eyes. The volunteers have to select from a list which emotion they think each face is expressing. The greater the number the volunteer gets correct, the higher is rated their emotional "empathy quotient." A second test is written. The volunteer is presented with around 60 statements and asked to give his or her agreement or disagreement with each with the same empathy objective as the picture test. I score below average on facial recognition and above average with textual empathy, illustrating the complexity and multi-facetness of Autism/AS, because images and text are processed by different parts of the brain.

Author's Note: In short; Aspies can't "read" people's faces, voices, body language and NTs can't read ours. That's what I term "The NT communication Gap" which leads to so much social mis or non-communication.

From the results of such tests and years of other extraordinarily detailed and deep scientific studies, Prof. Baron-Cohen has arrived at his startling twin theories, *The Empathy Systematizing Theory* (EST) and The *Extreme Male Brain Theory* (EMBT) that are connected closely with his Fetal Testosterone (FT) Theory to form an organic window into the world of an Aspie, whether male or female.

Firstly, it has long been established by a number of scientists, Baron-Cohen among them, that the *"Extreme Female Brain Theory* (EFBT) exists, (Baron-Cohen, S. (2003). *The essential difference: male and female brains and the truth about autism.* Such a person will be very empathic and caring towards the emotions, feelings and needs of others and will react to those exceptionally well, a care or aid worker perhaps, a kindergarten teacher or a nurse? All of which statistically trend toward being female-dominant characteristics and work specialisms. A possible reason for EFBT could be fetal exposure to excess Estrogen-the female hormone- in the womb.

During his and others' tests Baron-Cohen found that on average, males-regardless of Asperger's, age or culture -score lower on empathy tests than their female counterparts. He also found that Aspie males score lowest of all within their non-Aspie peer group and that Aspie females also display notably less empathy than their non- Aspie female counterparts. In fact, their scores closely resemble those of males, which is partly why Baron-Cohen has cited Asperger's Syndrome as producing the extreme male brain-in either gender. Aspies are not considered to be empaths, as we have discussed earlier. Baron-Cohen ascribes the Aspie brain development, again in either gender to excess embryonic exposure to Testosterone.

Empathy in Professor Baron's Cohen's work refers principally to the ability to interpret and relate to another person's feelings and situation. These emotions are usually expressed by voice tone, facial expression and body language. Aspies are not good at any of these skills which may explain our tendency towards being socially isolated. Aspies are frequently described as "loners" or "cold," at least by the media. That though is an over-simplification. The full reality is that although they do like their privacy and a low-stimulation environment more than most, few are loners by choice, but because of the sensory issues of social situations get sidelined by mainstream society. Some of us like to be alone at times, but nobody wants to be lonely

Furthermore, it must be made clear that the words "empathy," "sensitivity," "sympathy," and "compassion" are not synonyms and that Aspies are strongly capable of all those emotions. The great foundation set up by Bill and Melinda Gates is a case in point. Newton's famous love of animals and nature—he was the inventor of the cat-flap—and Van Gogh's compassion for the human condition are leading examples. My research findings are that Aspies have as much (or more) depth of emotional empathy as anyone else, but for different things and expressed in different ways. I think we have a different, deeper but narrower, not lesser emotional/empathy with different levels of deep empathy, compared with NTs. To paraphrase Shakespeare "we can love well, if not always wisely." (*Othello,* Act 5, Scene 2.)

On the other side of the Empathizing-Systematizing Theory, Baron Cohen and his team found that the lack of empathy is counter-balanced by an above average ability to systematize and that Aspies are the most systematic of all, again regardless of age or gender. "Systematic" in this context refers to the aptitude with which an individual analyzes, organizes, interprets and understands the operation of how systems, logic and processes work. Car mechanics, science, computer program writing, mathematics, surgery, and filmmaking are examples of systematics, in which traditionally at least, men do better than women. It also explains why many Aspies like possessions very ordered books set out in alphabetical order, clothes in certain places, and repetitive eating habits, etc.

To take computer programming, the process of creating algorithms is extremely detailed and systematic, the same with filmmaking and book writing. Aspies excel in each of those disciplines. Examples include Alfred Hitchcock, chemist Sir Henry Cavendish, Sir Isaac Newton, Jane Austen, and Thomas Edison. Facebook founder, Mark Zuckerberg is rumored to be an Aspie and Henry Ford was one. Chess-master Bobby Fischer, Abraham Lincoln, and the genius physicist and creator of the "Many Worlds Theory" of cosmology, Professor Hugh Everett III, all Aspies. Everett was also the father of the famous musician, Mark Everett, founder of the band *The Eels*.

Some of these Aspies we have already met, some are new friends, all of whom add ever more credibility to the theory.

All Aspie geniuses and those with ADHD/ADD have one thing in common: it's as if they have multiple-level programs running independently, but interactively in their minds at the same time. Each is brilliant at more than one thing (Polymathic) and is able to focus, often to the point of obsession on each in turn, often finding unseen connections between things, to create something entirely new. Those things may seem contradictory. Newton was a physicist, cosmologist, and mathematician, but also a Theologian and Alchemist. Leonardo was a painter, architect, military engineer, explorer, pioneer mapmaker and more, for all Aspies, though it is a continual desire to "connect the dots," to seek patterns and produce a greater revelation of what makes up the world, finding the order in its apparent chaos.

Albert Einstein's lifelong struggle to find the Grand Unified Theory (GUT) of physics: the equation which would balance the four/five? fundamental forces of The Universe is one example and a primary Aspie diagnostic criterion as well as being another reason why, like Leonardo, Aspies find completing projects so difficult. They get diverted easily, the "Minds like a butterfly" trap. It is something Aspies need to both recognize within themselves and address, as it's primarily their responsibility and problem and we need to face up to it and learn self-discipline. Without guidance that is next to impossible and all Autists can be extremely stubborn, infuriatingly so at times. Autists aren't saints by any stretch of the imagination, and being angry or despairing at them from time to time is natural and understandable. Autists get angry with each other too, it's all part of the human condition. No one is perfect and there is no shame in that.

Another Perspective:

There are naturally several theories about Autism/AS. To list them all would be a very lengthy and frequently repetitive task, as many are variations of each other to a greater or lesser extent. That is not so with the second major "stand alone" theory; *The Neanderthal Theory of Autism*. Neanderthals were so named after their first remains were uncovered in the Neander valley near Düsseldorf, in Germany. Over the last century, thanks to the hard, dedicated efforts by both individuals and groups in the fields of Archaeology in retrieving physical evidence of Mankind's past and forensic archaeologists for the scientific analysis of those finds, including the use of DNA sequencing and profiling techniques, we now have a fairly detailed, if still incomplete picture of humanity and its history.

Those individuals include Sir Arthur Evans who found the great palace of Knossos on the Greek isle of Crete, Gertrude Bell who uncovered much of our history and knowledge of ancient Jerusalem. Professor Heinrich Schliemann, discoverer of the legendary city of Troy in modern-day Turkey and the Spanish engineer Rocque Joaquin de Alcibierre who excavated the buried Roman city of Pompeii.

By combining their results and anecdotal evidence with that obtained by physicists, biophysicists, historians, and biochemists, science has achieved a new and clearer picture of the development and origins of us, modern humans (*homo sapiens*). It is somewhat different from what was thought until quite recently. Modern Man is currently considered to be only about 160,000-300,000 years old (*New Scientist,* June 11, 2003). Whichever end of that timeline is correct the fact is that at one point we and our genetically close cousins, Neanderthals co-existed across substantial regions of our planet for many tens of thousands of years. Their origins go back at least 600,000 years.

It was long thought that we caused the extinction of Neanderthals within a short time of meeting them.

Now though the latest archaeological and genetic information shows that not only did the two Man-types share land, but also sporadically interbred for tens of thousands of years, until only some 30,000 years ago, when Neanderthals suddenly and mysteriously disappeared (*National Geographic,* magazine, May 6, 2010). This idea of interbreeding was dismissed by the majority of scientists as lacking sufficient evidence. Then in March 2013 the skeleton of a child, a proven hybrid of human and Neanderthal was discovered in Northern Italy dating back about 40,000 years. The theory was then a proven fact, which more recent finds have confirmed.

The study was conducted by Prof. Ed Green and his team from the University of Santa Cruz in California and backed up a long-held belief by Anthropologists. This combination has given rise to the Neanderthal Theory of Autism. Some (but not all) of us to this day share somewhere between 1 and 4 percent of our DNA with Neanderthals. And, as we have seen with genetics, a little bit of cause may result in some very big effects, as we'll examine in the following chapter. Parts of that DNA, both regular and mitochondrial, contain many of the combinations which are now believed to be associated with Autism and especially Asperger's. It is found most commonly in specific ethnic groups, the most prominent being the Basques from an area straddling France and Spain.

To understand the potential of the theory it is necessary in the light of these recent discoveries to radically re-evaluate what Neanderthal man was really like, as compared with his previously "brutish" media-established public profile and how that may tie-in with Baron-Cohen's theories. Firstly, they had bigger brains and bodies than modern Man, (as did Cro-Magnons-size isn't everything. They were pale-skinned and often had reddish hair. Their extraordinary fine cave paintings pre-date ours by at least 4,000 years, as discovered by Dr. Alistair Pike of Bristol University in the UK, who found the oldest known cave art in El Castillo, Spain, dating back more than forty thousand years that is described in a Bristol University press release, June 14, 2012.

They invented complex games, played carved-bone musical instruments. They held elaborate burial ceremonies for their dead, complete with flowers, food, clothes, jewelry, and tools, which strongly suggests that they believed in an afterlife as strongly as the ancient Egyptians millennia later. They built permanent giant Mammoth bone-framed houses after previously being cave-dwellers (*The Daily Telegraph* December 18, 2011). Skeletal remains indicate they suffered from modern types of cancer and also that they could speak and would have done so with a high, slightly warbling voice-far removed from their media depiction as grunting savages. That warbling, sing-song voice is another very Aspie sign, as we know.

Neanderthals were wide-ranging hunters, using caves mainly as hunting lodges, but only rarely nomadic in lifestyle, unless external conditions forced it on them. That lifestyle would have made them very much in-tune with nature, both animals, plants and the seasons compared with the more gathering and then farming-based societies of Homo sapiens. They lived in small, family groups, as opposed to the more cosmopolitan and social Humans, who quickly learned to live in larger, settled communities, villages, towns and then cities. This would mean, in terms of evolution and the survival imperative that Neanderthal did not need the same degree of social and interpersonal skills which we take for granted today, but did need to be more aware of and "as one" with nature. Both of which are strongly Autistic and particularly Aspie traits, which may be significant clues in the makeup of the autism picture.

Like almost all non-human species of animal of whatever type, it is proposed that like Aspies, Neanderthals did not make frequent eye-contact with others, again unlike modern Man. Like their other contemporaries, us and Cro-Magnon-Man they used flint tools to cut wood, carve and to prepare meat and pelts for food and clothing. This also shows that they knew how to cook and shave and were therefore at least as intelligent and dexterous as ourselves at that time (*EarthSci*). Until 2010 it was assumed that they inhabited only the cold, northerly regions of Europe. Now though their remains have been found in Spain, France and modern Italy by a team from the University in Denver, Colorado. We can see that they, like us, were adaptable people.

Beyond that we know very little more about them. However, from their cave art and carving an intriguing observation has been made: its technique, application and composition were found to resemble very closely those of the modern Autistic/AS Savant artists, including Leonardo, adding further value to the Neanderthal-Autism theory.

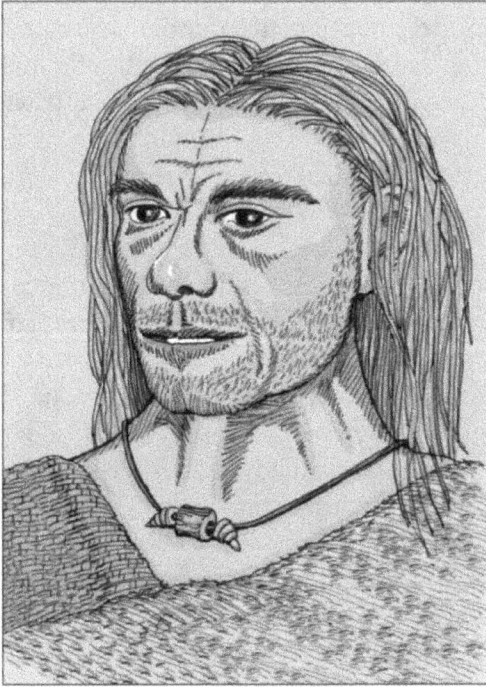

Neanderthal Man
ca. 600,000 bp

Image © Prof. David P Burkart

My DNA analysis has revealed a very high nearly 4% of Neanderthal DNA. As an experiment I set up with others re-sat the ARC's empathy-photograph test, yet with various animal faces chosen by random people from their own varied sources, books-magazines and photographs of animals in different situations: Happy, playful, in pain, aggressive, bored and so on, which were not revealed until after the test. They found pictures of dogs, horses, cats, fish, elephants, rabbits, birds, cows and many more.

For me and the majority of the other Aspies who scored below the average with human empathy, we scored well above average using Simon's criteria when the faces were those of animals. Of course, this only suggests an idea, because the sample size of people was too small to be truly scientifically valid. Still, it's nonetheless interesting, as more than 120 Aspies have now done it with nearly 67% reflecting a higher score with animal than with human images—very Neanderthal perhaps? It is definitely worth further investigation.

In over twenty-five years of professional experience, I have unquestionably seen that Autists/Aspies do display an unusual empathy, gentleness and affection for the natural world as a whole and animals in particular compared with many of their NT contemporaries. This love of and closeness to nature is an important and much undervalued quality in our current industrialized and polluted environment.

Author's Note: On the face of things this fact alone would seem, along with the artistic and religious depth of Neanderthals to put our two theories almost in complete opposition with each other, but perhaps that may not be the case at all. I believe they are both valuable pieces in an as yet incomplete picture of Asperger's.

This is my Theory:

Neanderthals being bigger and stronger than us must have possessed a more powerful endocrine system than our own, one able to produce at the very least the potency and volume of the growth hormones needed to achieve their size. It follows that it must be considered that they did the same for other hormones, including Testosterone in both genders. Part of the differences in their DNA and ours would account for that, maybe they had a sequence instruction or specific genes to "make lots of hormones." If, and it would be in very rare instances, the super testosterone-making code of that mechanism was inherited by a modern human, that would explain Prof. Baron-Cohen's FT theory in practice in a way that nothing else has or could.

148

Normally, in order for inherited genetic conditions to express in a child a copy of that gene from both parents is needed, hemophilia is an exception. Wilson's disease and Tay-Sachs are just two of the common Autosomal recessive conditions which do require a copy from each parent. Suppose that Asperger's is in that category and that both parents would need the right Neanderthal copies to produce the unusually high FT levels pivotal to Prof. Baron-Cohen's theory? Such a situation would confirm his theory and explain why Asperger's is so uncommon. If it took only one parent with the right Neanderthal DNA to produce high FT levels, that would be an even more unlikely circumstance, but the theory would remain intact, because Asperger's is very rare.

As we already know, just the presence of any particular genes do not guarantee their expression. Perhaps for even the minority with the right Neanderthal DNA it normally remains dormant.....for whatever reasons, unless it is "triggered" by some as yet unknown factor(s)—perhaps by some environmental fluctuation. It seems that there are quite a few combinations which would synergize both theories and in so doing greatly expand both our knowledge and assumptions to date.

It is research which needs to be done, not only for AS, but to increase our understanding of our past and the workings of our human Genome in general.

****

Psychological Fact: All people dream during sleep whether they remember the dreams or not and that includes blind people. These fall into two categories broadly: those who were born blind (congenital blindness) or became blind very young and those who lose their sight at a later stage of life, typically after the age of 5. The dreams of the young-blind contain only a very few and indistinct images, but a magical, subtle rainbow of sounds. The later-blind dream has much the same image intensity as the normally sighted and with only a little sound enhancement. This relates to autism as a "whole body condition" by again showing us how delicate the interaction between the physical and the mental really is. That fact alone should make us again ask searching questions about how we define, perceive and interpret that relationship in modern psychiatric and education practice.

Chapter 14: The Savant Syndrome

Savant (a French word) meaning a person of great wisdom or one with a special or unusual skill. A child born savant is also sometimes known as a "Child prodigy" who is well ahead, at least intellectually, of his/her peers, from a very early age, as Mozart was.

"Rain Man": The 1988 movie by Barry Levinson was based closely on a real, savant boy who became a legend. Kim Peek was born in 1951 and was misdiagnosed with severe autism. It was later found he had the rare genetic condition-F-G Syndrome, which caused his brain to be very different from normal. F-G syndrome is not an autistic condition. He remembered every word, date and time of anything. He memorized every book he ever read—over 12,000.

He could be given a random date, say 12/9/70 and immediately say what day of the week it was (a Saturday) for instance. He could do the same with addresses, telephone numbers or car plates. He read the 2 pages of a book at the same time-one with each eye, just staggering. Yet his measured IQ was only 87.

Tommy McHugh was a builder in Liverpool, England, a huge man with a criminal record for anti-social behavior and violence....until he suffered two brain hemorrhages after a fall in his bathroom in 2001. Surgeons struggled to save his life, finally he was discharged from hospital—a completely changed man in many ways, one of which was that he had forgotten both why and how to eat and walk, as well as his name.

Yet, with help he recovered. He acquired the reputation as a gentle giant from then on and began increasingly to display a brilliant and all-consuming passion for painting, of which no hint was ever present before the accident and that became his whole life and the source of a successful living. He had real talent and verve and taught himself the rest. After several internationally acclaimed art exhibitions, he died in 2012, aged 62.

Another "Acquired" savant with a similar story is Jason Padgett. Padgett did poorly at school in all subjects except sports and was a self-confessed "party boy." After leaving school he became a furniture salesman in Washington…until in 2002 he was badly beaten up outside a Karaoke bar. He suffered brain injuries and PTSD. Later fMRI scans showed the changes the assault had made to the left side of his brain. Over the next few weeks, he became a math genius' seeing complex math in his mind as geometric shapes-one of only about 20 cases ever known. He is now studying higher math.

The unusual experience of surgeon Dr. Anthony Cicoria is a similar story. He was born in 1952 and is now the chief of Medical Staff and Chief of Orthopedic Surgery at Chenango Memorial Hospital, Norwich, New York. Dr. Cicoria was struck by lightning in 1994 while standing next to an outdoor telephone booth. He was badly burned and his heart stopped—he needed resuscitation—luckily a trained nurse was standing just behind him. He was taken to hospital and quickly released, although he was feeling energy-drained and had difficulty in remembering things. So, he saw a neurologist, who could find nothing wrong. A few weeks later, Dr. Cicoria began to develop an interest in playing and listening to the piano to a near obsessive degree.

He bought one and taught himself to both play and compose within three months of the accident. He noted that his head seemed full of music, to which he devoted every spare moment. A very successful parallel career as a pianist/composer began in Vermont in 2007; his skills and fame continue to grow. He has now produced many CD's and can be appreciated on YouTube. Until being electrocuted, the Doctor had shown no noticeable interest in or talent for music.

A similar lightning-strike incident happened in August 1800 to a slow and sickly baby girl born in the small coastal town of Lyme

Regis, in Dorset, England. The child's name was Mary Anning, who from that moment onwards became strong and clever. She went on to become world famous as the "Mother of modern Paleontology"—the greatest and most successful fossil-hunter and recordist who has ever lived.

In 2010 the British Royal Society honored her memory by including her in its list of the top ten British women who have most influenced the history of science.

Born severely autistic, Stephen Wilshire from London, England was sent to a Special Needs School, where having previously been unable to speak he uttered his first word at the age of nine. He is now one of the world's greatest line draughtsman. He can look at any object, person, land or cityscape once and reproduce it on paper exactly, that has given rise to his nickname, "The human camera."

Savantism sheds important light across all areas of Neurodiversity. Firstly, it can be from birth, like classical autism, or acquired from brain damage later, like non-classical autism/NLDs. Secondly, it is far more common in men than women; and finally, it illustrates that high IQ is not necessary to having an exceptional gift, proving again the importance and potential of every single person and the respect each of us deserves.

Chapter 15: The "Whole Body Condition"

This chapter is about the nature of neurodiversity and how it can be interpreted to everyone's increased advantage and comfort. We know that its principle visible effects are in the social-cognitive field and beyond from the Autism Family Tree. Also that its less obvious results extend far further to affect the whole body and mind in a myriad of different ways, subtle and otherwise. The absolute cornerstone in the true understanding of Autism/AS is to realize that it is primarily a physical condition, not a mental one. The observed psychological presentations are caused by genetic structural variations in the brain, which also affect the rest of the body. That is why there are the distinct physical conditions associated with it, such as gut and stomach problems, Tuberous Sclerosis and Fragile X Syndrome- are just some of the *Co-morbid* conditions on our Tree. These apply whether autism is inherited or acquired later in life. If we can treat these core physical symptoms, social-cognitive ability always improves. This has been shown, time and time again. Of course, a person is more outgoing, happy and concentrates better if they sleep well, eat well and are not in pain. THAT is MY core "shout-out" message to doctors—and it didn't need an MD to say it!

That is perhaps the most important point this book seeks to make. Those with ASDs experience life completely differently from the NT community and that society's approach and attitude to Autism in all its forms needs to both change and expand in order to take full account of that truth. Anyone who says, "I understand," unless they are ASD simply can't and doesn't, and good specialist ND Doctors and Psychologists are hard to find.

Many Autists see life as a series of individual separate pages, rather than a continuous "work in progress"; building up a library of knowledge to be applied or recalled later, as required. This is why we tend to be naive and easily exploited, frequently repeating certain types of mistakes, notably emotional and financial ones.

Some have phenomenal memories, leading others to believe that Autists frequently make things up.

Many of us are very imaginative and creative, again leading to being disbelieved and the input under-appreciated or not understood at all. This type of rejection dogged Prof. Everett for much of his career. He was simply "too far ahead of his time" and a whole generation had to pass before his theories were understood and taken seriously, a situation which naturally made him depressed and led him to bouts of alcoholism and an early death at the age of 51. It's not too strong to say that society's ignorance and attitude was directly responsible for Everett's early death and furthermore again illustrates the fine line between physical and emotional wellbeing.

Even further proof of the nature of the "whole body condition" lies in the basic philosophy of modern medical practice, namely Evidence Based Medicine (EBM). It dates back about 150 years.

The idea is that clinical and psychological "Best Practice" is evolved by taking as much evidence from statistics, respectable publications and studies from around the world as possible to make a sort of *ad hoc* manual of the best and most successful approaches and treatment for each patient with any specific condition. The WHO provide us with an extensive guide, "World Best Practice," (WBP) based on their findings and the EBM philosophy.

There are, unfortunately, a number of conflicts inherent in this system of which we need to be aware. One is in the selection and quality of the "evidence" itself, some of which may be deliberately falsified, as in the Wakefield case, and, more recently by the revelation that certain Big Parma companies have simply paid researchers to make up the results they want in order to get drugs approved and marketed. **Another increasing problem is when good medical science contradicts current political and/or social fashions.** Other good evidence may be overlooked or misunderstood due to ignorance.

For example, the majority of evidence on Autism comes from males only, resulting in unbalanced practice failing to diagnose or misdiagnosis of females. Some evidence may simply be wrong and some omitted because of the financial implications of carrying out WBP are politically unacceptable due to cost-the reality of the infamous "profit before people" culture-whether in private or State healthcare provision. The best advice to all patients and carers is to research your regional policies, record them thoroughly and ask doctors lots of questions. Good doctors are always happy to answer; bad ones will refuse or be evasive.

One example of a failing in EBM practice stems from the differences of opinion on which evidence is used, and which is ignored and from when and where. The WHO sets the correct precedents by continually updating its advice as the latest findings emerge once they are verified. The same applies to the Life Extension Foundation of Fort Lauderdale, Florida, a non-profit organization, whose research; practice and positive contribution to good health worldwide cannot be praised too highly. It was started by Saul Kent and William Falcon in 1980 and now ranks as one of the finest and most accessible medical institutes in the world with a virtual "Who's Who" of top clinicians being actively involved. I recommend all their publications to anyone with an interest in personal or public health.

To give an illustration of this potential divergence of WBP from EBM we need only look at the question of how "acceptable" Blood test ranges differ from country to country, even some of those with clinically advanced facilities. This is because there is no one enforceable standard which the evidence in EBM has to meet. If the evidence upon which any particular region or country is basing their practice is wrong or outdated the whole process of EBM theory works against and not for the patient. There are still systems which use ranges outdated by more than 70 years when assessing blood, hormones, allergy/food intolerance, and pathogen (germ) tests, the UK being an example.

These old ranges were designed as "a healthy minimum" meaning in cold, cynical terms that the patient was just functional enough to work, not that he/she was in good health. The same is true of other diagnostic shortcuts. X-rays for example are used for cheapness where MRI or PET scanning provides better, more detailed information and as a result a better outcome for the patient. The spurious justification is, "we've been using X-rays for over a hundred years." On that argument practitioners should (and actually still do in some Practices) withhold life-saving medicines because they are deemed "too new," or not use anesthetics when performing operations, like 300 years ago, crazy thinking.

The same, sadly, is true of quality of diagnosis and response to Autism.

"Correct practice would be to base all test ranges for any population on the readings from its elite athletes. Doing this would force the medical sector to improve overall health by spurring them to treat ambitiously up to the highest standard not down to the lowest cost". It is a continuing scandal that in certain wealthy countries ordinary people are still denied basic life-saving and life-enhancing care on grounds of cost and any doctor who accedes to such a situation is by definition "unfit to practice" and should be criminally liable, as well as losing their medical license (I. Hale).

Author's note: Types of doctors to avoid—and there are a few:
The first is "Dr. Backhander" he/she is delighted to accept cash, holiday vouchers, goods and other "services", including sex, from certain unscrupulous drug companies in return for advocating and prescribing their products, irrespective of patient need or safety.

Then there is perhaps the worst type of all practitioners: "Dr./Nurse Ego." Those with the attitude, consciously or unconsciously, that medical/psychological progress reached its peak the day they got their diploma and could progress no further. They never bother to upgrade their skills or knowledge. You find these fossils of various ages, dotted right across the medical landscape; killing and failing as many patients and families today through arrogance and laziness as their predecessors did a century ago. The best advice is to "look, listen and learn" and always seeks a second opinion if possible. Look at the practice or hospital- does it seem clean, modern and motivated? Listen to other patients and carers' experiences. Research and learn both about the doctor and the medical issues with which you're concerned, again from textbooks, journals, or high-quality internet sites with PubMed, the LEF, and WebMD being among the best. The majority of doctors are of course good, so it is worth taking the time to spot the bad ones. The same point applies to clinics, hospitals and the psychiatric sector.

Important Autistic/Aspie Fact: Auties and Aspies do not return "normal" clinical test-range results. Our bodies are different, especially in the areas of yeast infection (Candida) allergies and food intolerance response, all of which point toward underlying autoimmune conditions. Those conditions are when the person's immune system attacks its own healthy cells instead of external pathogens. Rheumatoid Arthritis being one such condition, as well as the more Autism-specific ones. Allergies and Autism are both linked to an increased risk of migraines (Mayo Clinic). It is vital to find a specialist who understands and can properly interpret results correctly (*Autismtoday*.com, July-August 2004, Shaw, W).

The same principle applies to other areas: "normal" body temperature being one. It differs between some Auties/AS and NTs and your physician should be aware of this. It is this type of newly emerging evidence which again highlights Autism as a "whole body condition."

It is vital for Autists and AS people to be "drug and substance-aware" as well as food aware, as we may react differently from the average person. Some Aspies can't tolerate common prescription (and non-prescription) meds. Some need higher or lower doses of what they can tolerate, making it yet more important to have an informed practitioner because Aspies frequently "self-medicate" with a variety of things, legal or illegal. They are looking for "the normal" "to fit in," for coping strategies or at least some temporary peace of body and mind.

On the subject of drugs and the general population, it is poor practice that some doctors give out "one size fits all" dosages. 1000mg a day of drug Y may be fine for a 200 lb. 40-year-old male but is likely to prove an overdose for a 110 lb. 18-year-old female. Often adverse reactions, failures, and side effects stem from thoughtless mis-dosing, despite the drug company's often very specific and detailed guidelines to doctors. The hospital practice of prescribing by age, gender, and grams/milligrams per kilo, per patient is the proper, safer practice.

Returning to one of this book's early points, autistic people process their inner as well as their outer world very differently from the NT majority as Einstein among others explained. Auties/AS do not see color, taste food, hear, feel emotion, sense, speak or touch as others do. Some of these things they may do better or worse or just differently from the normal.

Take Einstein's brain, which he donated to medical research in his Will. Within a few hours of his death in April 1955 a pathologist had removed and dissected it into 240 cubes, taking hundreds of photographs while he worked, many unpublished until recently and now partially digitally reconstructed.

These images have now been made available and provide compelling evidence about the nature of both autism and genius. Firstly, size is not important. Einstein's brain was a little smaller than average, however its physical structure, even what we have seen so far was very different from "normal." He showed as we would expect marked differences. These included more complex synapses, especially in the prefrontal area which is crucial for thinking and spatial perception. The closeness and pattern of folding was very different from normal...and much more.

He could construct concepts and pictures in his imagination which others could not.

The same can be said of another, but NOT autistic Savant, Dr. Temple Grandin, whose brain, it has been revealed by tests and scans published in 2012, is both larger, especially in the left lobe (which ties in neatly with Dr. Cahill's brain findings at Irvine) than average and is quite structurally different in many ways from normal. Furthermore, her actual electro-chemical connections, "the wiring" of her brain is unusual as are her extraordinary abilities in the fields of reading, memory, spelling, pure thinking, sense of space, and logical reasoning.

She is a professor at Colorado University; a Doctor of Animal Sciences and Behavior, a famous inventor, and author of *The Learning Style* for people with autism, 1995 among many other publications. She is also left-handed and was the first real advocate and standard-bearer for Autists worldwide and for early diagnosis and interventional approaches to maximize the life potential of Autists and Aspies everywhere as well as a strong autism rights champion.

She also has weaknesses; predictably in the social/emotional sides of life, which are again explained by her unusual brain, where areas and connections associated with emotion and the ability to identify faces and facial expressions are weak by comparison with the average. Dr. Grandin is also the subject of the TV movie *Temple Grandin* (2010) starring Golden Globe-winning actress, Claire Danes.

For further strong scientific evidence towards understanding the nature of the Whole Body Condition we need to take a closer look at the various types of imaging and brain function monitoring techniques now available, some of which were used in Dr. Grandin's case because they help reveal the intricacies and workings of the human mind both in its NT and ND forms. The most common form of imaging is the old X-ray method; the earliest form of so-called "nuclear medicine" as it relies entirely on radioactive waves penetrating the body to form the picture. However, it produces only two dimensional results, which although fine for detecting broken bones and foreign objects, lack the detail, depth and resolution necessary for accurate situational analysis.

Its more complex successor is the CT (Computerized Tomography), machine that fires multi-directional X-rays from all round the patient simultaneously in "slices, which can vary in thickness down to 1mm for fine detail. These slices are then digitally reassembled by a computer to produce detailed 3-dimensional views that are a huge aid in all branches of medicine.

For scanning complex organs like the liver, stomach, or brain, "contrast CTs" may be ordered. In this procedure a type of dye is injected into the patient before the scan to highlight the area(s) under investigation for even greater accuracy and resolution. CT scanning is the most popular form of advanced non-invasive investigation because despite its disadvantages it is highly effective and a lot cheaper than the alternative not just in operation but in terms of the initial cost of the equipment. That said, with its inherent dangers I cannot fully endorse their use where a better option is available. The principal concern is that people tend to need a number of scans—regardless of the type used—and each PET/CT scan contains approximately the same level of radiation as 500 or more conventional X-rays leading to an increased risk of cancer developing in patients who need frequent scans. The second potential hazard is that some patients may develop anaphylactic shock as a reaction to the contrast material, although this is rare because good hospitals carry out thorough pre-scan tests.

A better and inevitably much more expensive method is the fMRI scan, using similar computer tomography but with magnetic waves instead of X-rays, they are not cancer-causers and because they differentiate better between hard and soft tissue like bone or muscle—again building a 3D picture in slices (something akin to the way the seabed is mapped by SONAR)—they provide a sharper, higher quality picture of the area being scanned, making them particularly useful for brain imaging.

In both types of scan the person lies very still in a kind of large noisy plastic-metal cigar tube, that can be very claustrophobic. Some people find it easier to have a small dose of a tranquillizer, usually Diazepam before having a scan, which also helps them remain motionless throughout the process, which is hard to do, but necessary for the best results. Scans can seem frightening, especially for young children, but there is nothing to fear when they are done properly by a good hospital or clinic. As with CTs a contrast material can be used for even greater resolution (with the same risk) but is needed less often, safeguarding more patients.

Many modern hospitals now provide ear defenders to cancel the noise and a pleasant projected view inside the machine to reduce anxiety. Typically, the view is a summer field and calming music accompanies it. This is especially good with children, who may also get their favorite cartoons as a reward during and after the scan.

These scanning techniques have revolutionized our understanding of the brain and have given us unimpeachable evidence that the structure and operational method of the autistic/AS brain is quantifiably different from non-autistic ones. This has been re-confirmed using an even more modern technique, the functional-MRI (f- MRI). This allows the actual blood flow to the brain to be watched in real-time and in color. The procedure itself is the same as the standard MRI, except that a unique contrast material is used. By observing blood flow, it shows which areas of the brain are most activated by what kind of stimulus. Combined with EEG (Brainwave) monitoring they give us a very clear working map of where everything is and what it all does, for instance the center which processes sight.

An EEG-an Electroencephalograph monitors and records the electrical activity in the brain-the brain receives information, processes it and gives the appropriate responses by means of bio-chemically generated electrical signals-we are electric beings. To understand the idea, it is worth thinking of the brain, human or animal as a kind of electro-chemically etched-(imprinted) 4D multi-layer, squidgy (im) printed-circuit board. :) Alternatively, we can compare the brain with an old-fashioned telephone exchange, where Autistic brains connect differently from NT ones.

By following the electric current, we can see which stimuli produce which results in any part of the brain, images, music, smells, movement and so on. Autistic brains display different electrical "maps" from those of NTs.

Each time we experience or learn something it forms a new etched physical pathway on the brain, that is the "soft wiring" of the brain. Those etched paths are called "Engrams." That applies equally to good and bad experiences. The earlier in life and more intense the experience, the quicker and more entrenched the memory (Etching) will be. These neuron (transmitter electro-chemicals) pathways form easiest while we are young, enabling children to learn things very fast, languages being one important example. On the dark side it is also why childhood traumas can be so life-dominating. By constantly re-enforcing certain behaviors we deepen and sharpen those pathways. That's how learning works, why "practice makes perfect" and why therefore positive learning is so important. It also explains why people get "stuck in their ways" as they get older, by constant repetition of routine behaviors.

To avoid this, constantly seeking new hobbies and challenges like doing an online course, going to the gym, or playing video games help keep the faculties intact and lively. The brain needs exercise as much as the body. "Engrams" and the junctions where they interconnect and relay messages (like roundabouts) are the Synapses. Knowing this, it is possible by various methods some of which we shall outline in the final chapter to re-program the brain to more positive operating patterns.

Brain Fact: Left or right brain dominance: All of us have the two hemispheres (sides) to our brain and one is always dominant. The strengths given by the left brain lie in the areas of logic, math, reasoning, planning, analytic thinking and languages. Those who favor the right are better at recognizing people, have better social and interpersonal skills, a greater appreciation of art, color and music and tend to be more intuitive and creative. The author has been tested and is very left-brain dominant. Again, this agrees with the idea that AS at least reflects structural differences from normal in the left forebrain region. I strongly believe and assert that Autism/AS is not a simple pathological state, but an entire "State of physical being and mental Consciousness," unique in itself and should be appreciated as that.

Chapter 16: Help is at Hand

So, what can we do? In addition to the strategies already detailed, fortunately for many but not all Autists, the answer is "quite a lot"- in fact too much to fit into this guide- but here are a few paths worth exploring. The most important of which are effort, understanding and patience on top of some of the therapies already mentioned like hypnosis, drug treatment, clinical testing assessments, dance and music. **The Golden rule is "Force Never! Encourage Forever." (I. Hale)**

Omega 3 Fish oil is good for everyone. For a fully grown adult the useful amount is approximately 6 mg per pound of body weight (about 1200mg) per day. For a child under 16, half that. Fish oils act as blood thinners; so anyone on prescribed blood thinners should consult their doctor first. But the big point is that studies have shown Omega 3 to be beneficial for some childhood autism and Depression *(Biol Psychiatry.* 2007 Feb 15; 61(4):551-3), as well as helping to keep arteries clearer of plaques, lessening the risk of some cancers, heart disease and Dementia, reducing acne, inflammation in general (including in the gut) and arthritis in particular among many other benefits. It is a supplement I use daily along with Vitamin E and Chamomile or Green tea.

Nootropics: a.k.a. "Smart drugs" and supplements. A whole new generation of drugs and supplements, some derived from natural ingredients, others laboratory made, which nourish the natural chemicals of the brain, improving memory, speed of thought and intelligence. These are applicable to everyone. They are still mostly first-generation preparations and their long-term benefits/hazards are as yet not known. Current popular ones are L-Carnitine, Vitamin B and K groups, Vitamin D, 5-HTP, SAM-e, DHEA, Piracetam, Modafinil, CDP-Choline, Adderall, Mito CO Q10, and Folic Acid, to name just a few.

Separately, there are being developed electronic devices that could, if they succeed, control brainwave activity to avoid over stimulation and produce the calm level waves. They would end meltdowns and epilepsy forever. They are the Neuro-equivalent of a heart pacemaker. Others are planned to hugely increase IQ. It will be worth checking closely on their progress over the years ahead through the work of the Transhumanist Movement and "Biohackers." (Lee, 2019) It all sounds very Sci-fi, but it's real and it's happening now. The potential is certainly exciting and hopeful.

Returning again to education practice, Ruth Wilson's book *Special Educational Needs in the Early Years* (Wilson, 2003) is excellent, covering in a comprehensive manner most of the current SEN methods, both for the school and at home. She emphasizes the positive role of learning by play, especially outdoor provision to encourage social skills and interaction with other children and the environment. In this structure, the teacher sets up the situation then praises the child at suitable moments when they display positive behavior. By these actions, positive behavior is re-enforced at the earliest stages of development. She points out the need for teachers and social services to encourage parents to continue this method at home. I have found through my own practice that this method is very effective, with the *caveat* that it is also very demanding both in terms of teacher training, time, concentration and in requiring the very low pupil-teacher ratio already stated in order to be effective.

A second notable point Wilson makes, is how vital it is to provide "Quiet Rooms" or "Time Out Spaces." Autistics are easily upset by the brain being overloaded by stimuli-physical or mental and either shutting down, or having a meltdown and over-reacting by lashing out, usually verbally but sometimes physically as all teachers know. To have a facility that allows them to calm down in a safe place and recover is very helpful. If the space can provide quiet, soothing music and low light, then so much the better. This can take the form of a refuge room away from the demands of the classroom or home and works better than anything else, including drugs in my experience of SEN groups in various settings. It must be clear that such rooms are left open as an opportunity for the child, not locked as some sick kind of punishment cell, which will only make the child more shut in and traumatized than he/she already is.

In similar vein from the University of Mysore in India is Dr. S Venkatesan's *Children with Developmental Difficulties* (Venkatesan, 2004). It is a catalogue of practices, more systematic than Wilson's and containing less commentary and professional anecdotes. At this point, it is worth remembering that not all children with developmental difficulties are Autistic, Downs's children are another example, but most SEN methods are equally applicable to all physically able groups. He advocates teaching by small increments of success in a very carefully structured program, a multi-step process aimed at skills acquisition.

He calls his system **"Short Term Goal Teaching**." The idea is based on the fact that these children have concentration difficulties, particularly those with ADHD. So he builds skills, block by block, one small step at a time. He has devised a series of techniques for promoting attention and concentration. He describes one such... "For older children, number game activities like forward repetition of digits, presented by the caregiver/teacher at the rate of one number per second, can be carried out to improve concentration." Another one is the learning of three-word sentences by constant repetition both spoken and written. However, like Wilson he too stresses the importance of the family/caregivers in maintaining the system at home. Dr. Venkatesan's reputation for success is outstanding.

There are two themes in common with these authors and others, namely, the agreement in the imperative of early diagnosis to maximize the best results and the stressing of the paramount importance of the role and attitude of each child's home environment-the parents or caregivers.

Another big inspiration for this guide in educational terms was Philip Kendall's *Childhood Disorders* (Psychology Press, 2000). In it he alphabetically lists each condition and describes its causes and presentations and again the central role in children's lives which parents and other family members involved in the situation or treatment can play. Instead of working one-to-one with child therapists he often chooses to spend at least some time teaching the "parents to work with the child" Not only should we care about the autistic, but also about their supporters. It is they who, in combination with teachers, predict the child's future. It must be emphasized on top of this that the first duty of any caregiver in whatever circumstance is to care for and inform themselves—otherwise they will fail.

A teaching method I have used successfully for SEN children is Kinesthetic activity-based "play teaching," based on Professor Howard Gardner's theories of multiple types of intelligence that were further developed by Dr. V Prakash again, at Mysore University. Kinesthetic learning is a teaching and learning style in which learning takes place while the student actually carries out a physical activity, rather than passively sitting at a desk, listening to a lecture or watching a demonstration/video. Following on from the "learning through movement" method is the idea of learning through dance, joining a drama group, photography classes, nature-walks or singing Karaoke. Each is great for the mind, the body, and their ability to build and enhance positive social interactions and patterns. I sing Karaoke and find it very stress-relieving and confidence-boosting—debatable whether it has the same effect on the audience though. :)

Bodily Kinesthetic Intelligence is the ability to use the body to express emotion (as in dance and body language) and to play games. Autists are naturally given the chance—playful and keen to create a new product (such as crafts and invention). By interacting with the space around them, students are able to learn, remember and process information more readily. In fact, the body instinctively knows and can learn many things which our conscious minds do not and cannot know in any other way. It's called "muscle memory" and is part of every person's array of often untapped talent, whether Autistic or NT. For example, it is how our bodies learn to type, ride a bicycle, stitch a cloth, or ice-skate.

My experiences using either Kinesthetic or music teaching have been very successful—and when combined they are the best system there is—not only from an academic perspective things like learning to count, but also for physical health and inner calm. My thing is a combination of Mozart or Mahler with balloons or beanbags according to the type of group and their age/disability. People bat balloons or play "catch" with beanbags while listening to Mozart AND doing the learning exercise, all at the same time. An example would be reciting math tables or learning a poem.

It is a technique which works almost as well on adults. Playing Mozart helps them conquer exam nerves as well as revise and recall facts more effectively prior to exams or tests-even the driving test. I have done the same thing at business seminars-beanbags and Mahler, helps in life/career, business or goal coaching. It is fun and is a great team-building exercise as well.

Learning with the use of flashcards, shown at one second intervals, imparts knowledge virtually unconsciously. This fascinating synergy between the conscious and the unconscious is an area that psychologists have investigated since Freud. The brain alone is not the whole story. Consequently, many students do best while being able to move around and interact with their surroundings, boosting their creativity. People tend to lose concentration if there is little or no external stimulus going on. It is useful to employ activities and games which challenge hand-eye co-ordination, and some well-supervised indoor sports like table tennis, handball, and especially swimming. Swimming is the complete whole mind and body workout making it perfect for Autists and Aspies alike...and you too.

When the brain is challenged it produces increased electro-chemical activity, which in turn aids memory. Incorporating one or more of the above-mentioned activities into lessons helps children to take part more completely in the activity and remember the lesson more clearly. For instance, an early exercise would be for two students to face each other and hit a balloon back and forth as quickly as possible with their hands while practicing the alphabet, each student takes a turn saying a letter or word at the instant of hitting the balloon. After practicing that way, the students next use their elbow to hit the balloon as they say the letter. Later, to make it even more challenging the students use their non-dominant elbow, knee or hand to hit the balloon or catch the beanbag. Doing that helps to develop that side of the brain, making the person more complete and balanced. This exercise is an excellent tool. It can be used for learning such things as counting, the days of the week, the months, naming fruits, vegetables, flowers, telling the time, learning phrases, rhymes and sentences, which can be written on a board or overhead-projected to augment the "learn-by-eye" response. Kinesthetic exercises are excellent opportunities to discover, practice, and reinforce learning. They are best when kept simple and purposeful. If an exercise is too complicated students become bored or frustrated and will not learn well. The exercises should be short, well-spaced (only done a few times and not every day) approximately twenty minutes or less for each session and of course, they too, can be done at home.

From experience I will add that learning a musical instrument to any level of achievement as one of the best and most enjoyable things anyone can do, even banging two spoons together or strumming a banjo. Music is a fantastic combination of fun, increasing knowledge, helping dexterity, self-expression and a great all-round therapy. The most famous proponent perhaps was Albert Einstein with his violin. Learning music is knowledge in itself but it also increases the brain's overall fitness and capacities and as a result it will learn all the other things better as well. Learning to juggle gives a real boost to self-esteem and physical co-ordination, both of which are traditionally weak areas for Autists. Better still, all these activities tend to be in a group which aids their social and emotional development, they are all win-win activities. The secret again is to keep the sessions short enough to remain a joy and not become a chore.

Taking that a stage further brings us to the controversial topic of "The Mozart Effect." Good sounds (Sonics) and music particularly by Mozart are cited as the most beneficial. If prospective parents have any autistic genetic history (or even if they don't) ante-natal (before birth) exposure to Mozart for about twenty to thirty minutes twice a day is widely medically recommended. Studies have indicated that it stimulates and activates the vital P (perception) centers in the brain—perhaps increasing innate childhood intelligence by as much as 10% and aiding the ability to both learn and recall in later life. It certainly produces a strong feeling of well-being in mother and child and decreases depression, as well as the marked anxiety so prominent in most forms of Autism.

Pieces by the Austrian composer Gustav Mahler have been shown to act similarly and there may be others as yet undiscovered. The basic fact is that some music or sounds can be as calming, stimulating or healing as anything drugs without the risks. Sonics have been demonstrated to literally reprogram (by re-etching) the brain pathways in a positive fashion, in a similar but much healthier way as certain types of Behavioral modification, Psycho-active medications and other things do. The secret is to keep trying all the alternatives, initially one at a time and if necessary, in combination until you find the combination that works best for you and your child. It can be a long, hard process and I give no false hope or slick, easy promises. All I can say for sure is that Music has at times greatly helped me and many, many others, even though science can't yet fully explain how.

Painting, drawing and such activities as clay modelling and knitting are all tools of "Art Therapy" that are well-proven to help some people. The goal of art therapy is not so much to produce great or necessarily even realistic art but internally representative art, although some great artists have been discovered through it. Its real goals are to permit and enable non-verbal communication and emotional expression, to reveal the inner world to the outer one. This accomplishes important tasks, social interaction, trust, release, or explanation of distress- the idea that a picture can tell a thousand words. It can explain, not only in action but in technique and choice of colors a great deal about a person's past and present mental and emotional state, which helps psychologists find the best ways forward. People and not only Autists and especially the young find it less traumatic to show if they have been bullied or abused in some alternative, non-verbal way. This is so even to those who are able to do so, remembering that some Autists cannot process words and are unable to speak. This makes them particularly vulnerable and for them art therapy/communication can be a real life-saving way of communicating how they are.

Throughout the art sessions, the methods and media used can be both flexible and varied. Film/photography one day, painting by brush or fingers the next and perhaps a craft approach, pottery or sculpting after that. Some of history's greatest painters like Pablo Picasso and Joseph (WM) Turner frequently painted with their fingers for a more intense and immediate effect as well as to create different textures on the canvas and true 3D effects. The basic idea is to relieve, reveal and calm the mind. It works. Other helpful skills are learning Yoga and Meditation techniques-something I have never managed to do, but a lot of people do and report very positively on the effects for them, although some negative effects have been reported, including a loss of interest in day-to-day life. Hypnosis can induce a calm relaxed state of mind as can the use of Executive "Stress balls," and a good walk in the open air. Aromatherapy can help avoid the "Meltdowns" caused by the sheer sensory impact and pressures of modern life. Smell is, after all the most evocative of all the senses and the right ones are almost as effective as music in calming the mind.

Chapter 17: Why Do They Work?

The reason goes back to our look at the EEG machines which monitor the electrical activity of the brain through soft painless electrodes taped to the scalp. These reveal that the activity of the brain varies through five distinct frequencies or "brainwaves," much the same as radio stations do. In the brain these frequencies are Delta, Theta, Alpha, Beta and Gamma and each reflects the degree of excitation or relaxation of the person and is a different shaped wave from each of the others, (as shown below). Delta waves are the longest, slowest waves with a tone of around 0.1-3.9 Hertz (Hz) and indicate a deep state of sleep, Theta waves, 4-7.9 Hz are associated with the less deep periods of the normal 90 minute sleep-cycle as well as with states of deep meditation and hypnosis. Alpha waves, 8-13.9 Hz are when you're calm, relaxed and attentive, perhaps watching TV. Beta waves 14-25 Hz dominate when thinking, working, very aware, active or worried. Gamma waves 25-100Hz signify complex intellectual tasks, Chess, advanced mathematics or extreme situations and/or stress above 40Hz.

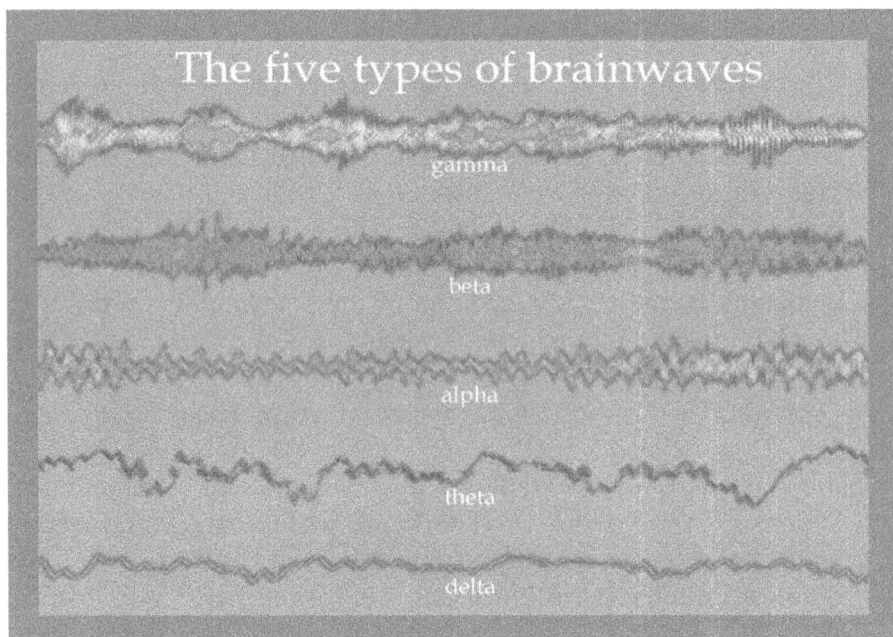

The five types of brainwaves

gamma

beta

alpha

theta

delta

The types of activities described above like art therapy help calm the brain from over-stimulation toward the more relaxed states where healing takes place. The brain's patterns are in reality more complex than set out here and each frequency has sub-frequencies all with their good and proper function, but if through stress, particularly with Autistic imbalance towards the more active frequencies continues for too long, "Meltdowns" or "Shutdowns" happen as the brain produces too much "noise" from too many contradictory rapid signals. HFAs, if not all Autists derive their creativity, hyper-ness, sleep problems and possibly a proportion of their gut problems from all this activity. Excess stress makes the body release the hormone Cortisol made in the adrenal glands sitting on top of each kidney. Cortisol makes us hyper and "ready-for-action" along with Adrenaline. It's released in threatening or exciting situations like sex or sport and usually returns to normal levels as soon as they've passed. However, if the exposure is prolonged without a break—"de-stressing"—it damages the immune system leaving some people (but not all) more prone to diseases like cancer, colds, stomach and gut lining issues. Calming things down helps readjust the balance and contributes towards achieving a stable, healthy and happy state of body and mind. It is this hormone which is largely responsible for PTSD.

Please encourage your Autist to learn a sign language, whether British or American (B/ASL). Both are internationally recognized non-verbal languages in their own right and learning grants are widely available. Some autistics/AS are poor verbal as well as non-verbal communicators and empowering them with another, essentially physical language greatly enhances their personal and social development well beyond anyone's expectations. There are those who can be poor listeners or in the case of Dyslexics, readers/writers. Learning by eye and touch rather than ear can prove far more effective than standard classroom techniques. Even better it increases their potential social opportunities to include that other special group, those who are deaf and have to sign, and, as a bonus it can provide an immensely rewarding and lucrative career for those able to deal with either the mainstream or a sheltered working environment.

Regarding employment conditions:

Employers may need to make provision for Autist/AS/Savant workers like quiet office space, lower light levels and if on a production line extra ear and tinted eye defenders. Gauze or other breathing masks reduce the chances of airborne irritants-dust, insects and pollen for outdoor workers and other allergy-causers for indoor ones. Gloves or suits/overalls do the same job, protecting the skin from harmful chemicals and other reactive materials, basically just small tweaks to normal health and safety codes in the workplace, along with flexible hours.

On the subject of employment, it is hard for Aspies and especially gifted ones to hold down steady, long-term jobs. Unstimulating work quickly gets boring and stressful, leading to confrontation or a sudden resignation, surprising everyone. Aspies "hold in" their feelings causing a build-up of tension until an apparently trivial incident ignites a strong reaction-one often misinterpreted as an overreaction. Aspies may not only frequently change jobs but also make several radical career changes during their working lives, looking for that elusive "right fit." In this currently hostile economic cycle that can quickly lead to periods of severe financial hardship, homelessness and the personal despair which goes with those. It is important for Aspies to have sound financial planning and advice, especially in the fields of savings, pensions, and insurance inculcated into them in order to insulate them against their natural restless, creative and sometimes unwittingly self-destructive life pattern. Ideally that process should begin at home as early as possible.

Sleep:

"For good health, make sleep a priority" wrote Lois E. Krahn, M.D. of the world-famous Mayo Clinic. She is right for Autists, NTs, young and old. Lack of sleep contributes to lowered immunity, impaired performance at work, relationship breakdowns, brain cell death, which can lead to full-blown NLD, Autism, psychosis, premature aging and not least dementia, as described in *The New Scientist* journal, September 24th, 2009. It aids the formation of the deadly plaques we have discussed, whereas the use of sleep drugs reduces it (Annals of Neurologoly, April, 2023)

While not suggesting sleeping pills- usually either hypnotics or sedatives- as first resort, if other things fail-use them and for as long as needed-under medical supervision. Do whatever it takes to get enough sleep at any age. Sleep is every bit as essential to a good life as food or water for the maintenance, regeneration and happiness of body and mind. That is equally true with regards to seniors' health. It is also a total long-standing myth that people need less sleep as they get older (Fred Cicetti, *Live Science*, 10 May 2009). The opposite is true; lack of sleep causes increasing disability, then death.

The minimum amount of sleep needed—except for a few, very rare genetic variant individuals like the late UK Prime Minister Margaret Thatcher—for an adult is 6 hours a night; for optimum wellbeing the target is 8-10 hours and for children and adolescents, a lot more. Today we average three hours sleep less per night than our nineteenth Century Ancestors, and are seeing more mental illnesses than ever as a direct result.

Even slight sleep deprivation causes tiredness (Lethargy), inability to learn and/or concentrate, unsafe driving, and bad temper.

How many children diagnosed with ADD/ADHD are simply the victims of an ignorant or deprived family situation? Those who are kept up or out to all hours by selfish parents or ones who do not care about their children's outside or online activities? Make no mistake at all: such irresponsible adult behavior is a form of child abuse and teachers should react accordingly if they suspect it by alerting Social Services. Also, how many totally normal children (or adults) are, along with their families, the victims of poverty and whose parents or partners are blameless due to impossible home (or homeless) circumstances? **How can a hungry child be expected to learn, for example?**

Because of the unusual brain structure and CNS activity, good regular sleep, especially during the rigid times demanded by modern industrialized nations- the night-is hard for Autist/AS people and made worse by their extra sensitivity to sounds, light, textures, allergies and so on. Many Autists are naturally nocturnal. On the positive side, that tendency gives some Autists the advantage of working the better-paying night shifts with comfort and efficiency, benefiting both them and the employer. They have to deal with less traffic and the night is quieter. Autistic night workers can be a very valuable asset as they will be sharp and alert at times when NT employees are flagging or dozing off. This perhaps relates to the Neanderthal Theory. Autists simply, in a sense, cannot belong comfortably in parts of the modern environment and need a simpler, more natural lifestyle to thrive.

An Autist child may sleep poorly or wake easily because of noises that their parents/caregivers can't hear. Always listen carefully to the child and act on what you are told. Sleep-deprivation explains many of the symptoms (like AD(H)D) experienced by both Autists. Actively involve the child in the construction of a good sleep environment and routine, explaining in detail what is being done and why. Aspies and HFAs in particular ask a lot of questions as parents and teachers may already know.

In a constantly noisy neighborhood white or pink noise machines work well. Non-toxic wadding, wood and old newspapers, wax or Silicone earplugs along with rubber wedges to dampen vibration provide a good alternative to expensive specialist soundproofing materials.

In addition, aircraft-style "sleep kits" of ear muffles, RED eye masks, and RED, heavy curtains to cut out sound and light, serve the same purpose.

Trust me, I've tried them all. The goal is to create a reassuring and reliable "sleep capsule" at a constant temperature of around 68F/20C for optimal effect. You have created something which can benefit everyone of any age, NT or not for years. The earplugs are reusable and should be washed every day. Silicone ones have the added advantage of gently easing out any excess earwax as well.

Another successful idea is to light the bedroom with low-level ambient red light (although for some people green works better). We don't know why it helps; it just does. Some have found that simply moving their bed round to face North (Head-end, South-feet) greatly improves their sleep. Others find a lavender pillow works; again no one has any idea why. "Box beds" are awesome and either ordered or easily made from standard **wooden** bedframes.

Under medical supervision consider the use of the hormone Melatonin.

These options help relax the child and by reducing anxiety in the short, medium and long term promote closer bonding from the extra trust created by success, bringing the child and the whole family closer together. Love, reassurance, expressing confidence, support, and tolerance are all essentials.

Parents and caregivers must though avoid excessive spoiling and over-protection-both perfectly natural reactions-but they hinder healthy development and can "infantilize" a child throughout his/her whole life, to the point where he/she will never attain their full adult potential. Any form of abuse will; and over-coddling is also a form of child abuse.

Overpraise for no or trivial performance is equally bad. It stunts the child's development and may create a Narcissistic personality which will be a heavy, dangerous and isolating burden in later life. We all wish, for our children at least, that the world is made of candy floss—but it isn't and it does nobody any favors to pretend otherwise. That "line" between, protecting, spoiling and abuse can be very narrow and very fuzzy at times. It will only be found with time and by trial and error because it varies with both changing circumstances and the natural personalities of the people and family traditions involved.

It is hard to do, accept that; take a deep breath and smile, if only at the irony of it all. Smiling alone, even if you don't mean, it causes the Endorphins in the brain to be released and you'll feel a bit better and less frustrated for a while, giving you the chance to relax and regroup.

Parents:

Please don't ever feel guilty about taking time out for yourselves every now and then-you're human, you deserve it, you need it and it'll help you in all sorts of subtle ways in the years ahead and help you to be a better carer. Guilt and resentment born of frustration and exhaustion can lead to anger and that is corrosive to any relationship. So have guilt-free respite days whenever you can.

Diet:

It's imperative for everyone to remember that Autism is not any kind of disease, mental or physical. It can't be caught person to person. It's not caused by a worm, or a parasite, nor an infection or fungus. It can be helped and any advantages maximized. To repeat: there is no "cure," whatever claims may be made.

There are also, as we've noted many branches to the Autism Family Tree as well as its Co-morbidities. Two very common ones are Crohn's and Celiac Disease, as well as other digressive complications. There are no completely verified global studies yet published to prove it, but recorded incidences by parents, Autists, Doctors, Specialists and teachers leave little question of their place in the tree. Both are serious, predominantly inherited conditions, that affect men and women about equally, but smokers have more than double the risk of Crohn's Disease than non-smokers. Both are autoimmune in origin and attack the whole gastrointestinal tract causing over time, severe pain, Rheumatoid arthritis, IBS, inflammation, nausea, rashes, eye problems, and the loss of the body's ability to absorb vital nutrients and vitamins from food. That results in bone loss, poor growth in children, depression, anemia and a host of other bad things. In severe untreated cases either condition can cause cancer or ulcers. These can eat through the gut wall and without emergency surgery to remove and repair the damaged portion, allow its contents to seep out into the thoracic cavity, leading to probable blood-poisoning (Septicemia) and death.

Both conditions first target the small intestine and in neither instance do doctors really understand their causes, but they differ in other ways. Celiac tends to present earlier in life, making diagnosis easier. Celiac patients don't normally run a fever and the two conditions although having a lot in common, including Autism; have different triggers. Celiac is triggered predominantly by the protein gluten, found in numerous things: bread, pasta, wheat, fried things, butter, cakes, soups, beer, and a whole lot more.

The top treatment for Celiac is a 100% gluten-free diet, but it doesn't always work without help.

Other treatments are common for both diseases. These are anti-inflammatory medications, steroids, painkillers and Immune system suppressing drugs to diminish the severity of the body's reaction to whatever it is intolerant to. For Crohn's, we don't know. Neither is curable, but they are, with careful lifestyle choices and specialist monitoring, usually manageable throughout life. Diagnosis is by blood and/or allergy testing, scans, and perhaps a gut biopsy in difficult cases. Whatever the result, identifying and reducing possible allergens reduces the impact of the disease. I counsel patients to have the full blood tests for allergies; airborne, waterborne, insect, plant, fungi and food and to undergo the "Scratch-test," where shallow scratches are made on the skin, usually on the back or upper arm and a suspected allergen is brushed on. If the skin erupts, it's another irritant to avoid. If not, it's OK. Pin and patch testing follow the same principle.

To save money, with great care and after medical instruction you can do your own scratch test at home. Disinfect your skin, wash, and then get a small blunt needle. Dip it in a suspected allergen, like bran and just white-graze (don't puncture) the skin. Wait 10 minutes to see if a red welt comes up, indicating a reaction. It's free and pretty accurate. The needle should be disinfected with boiling water after each test, but where a lack of facilities or money exists, it's a lot better than nothing. I have successfully experimented with it on myself a number of times to confirm both its safety and that it works.

Milk:

Cow's milk is the most common cause of irritation and intolerance because it is made for baby cows, not people. Firstly, at least 60% of all adults across the world cannot digest it and the figure is higher among all Asian communities (*USA Today*, August 30, 2009). It contains Lactose, an acidic sugar to which many people, myself included, have a sharp intolerance. Milk is high in Gluten, causing the problem with cakes, cheese and butter for celiac patients and fourthly virtually all animal milk has Casein in it, a Phosphoprotein used in paint-making-as well as ice-cream, pastries and other foodstuffs. Casein binds with gluten to cause the problem. It is the combination of the two which triggers the reaction. Those intolerance levels are high and can be very severe…and there is some, as yet inconclusive evidence tying its consumption to Autism and NLDs.

The Elimination Method:

This is an approach to reducing irritants which offers many advantages and a couple of disadvantages over other methods. It is free, thorough and very accurate, and if done carefully, riskless. The disadvantage is that it's very painstaking and time-consuming.

Basically, you note every single thing you eat, drink, or are otherwise exposed to—including household substances such as laundry liquid—over a month and then eliminate one at a time. This means NO exposure at all to it for 2-4 weeks. If you feel better, note the substance and avoid it; if not, it's safe for you. Then move on to the next one until the list of dos and don'ts is completed. It works but can take over a year to complete fully. Most people find that it's well worth it, because diet affects mood and consciousness, via the gut. By eliminating irritants Autistic conditions such as ADD/ADHD have been greatly improved and, in some people, almost completely stopped. On top of that, anything which helps improve physical health improves mental and emotional health as well. **"Get the body healthy first, then the mind will heal itself" (I. Hale).**

Epilogue

The principal reasons for writing this book were to answer some questions and provide more background and context to the subject.

The third and perhaps most important question I shall try to address now: American President John F Kennedy said, "What makes journalism so fascinating and biography so interesting is the struggle to answer that single question, 'What's he like'?" (Ben Bradlee *Conversations with Kennedy*, WW Norton, 1984) That's the big question I try to answer from both my professional and personal Autism perspective…"what's it like?"

Well…it's very much like living in a moving greenhouse, isolating. The greater the extent of the Autism, the thicker and darker the glass and the tighter the windows and door are sealed. We can see out and hear you, as you can us, but most of the time it is distorted, sometimes physically, always emotionally and often "out of step with others." It's like watching a movie with the dialogue out-of-synch with the picture or hearing a language you know but in an unknown accent. You understand-and you don't fully understand or misunderstand at the same time- there's gap somewhere. You're not sure if it's their "language" that's wrong or yours. It is by turn a frustrating, sometimes frightening and frequently confusing situation for everyone. And…because people don't understand and expect a person to "get over it," or "learn to cope better", neither of which are possible, it only gets harder as the person gets older and becomes ever more marginalized and their needs increasingly ignored. We almost literally become invisible in society as our parents and support fall away.

There is no doubt that knowledge about Neuro-diversity, notably clinical understanding, has as I predicted in the previous edition improved and expanded greatly in the intervening years.

Society too has become less harsh; at all age group levels we celebrate this progress. Sadly though, provision and support for us in education, in housing, and worst of all, early diagnosis has gone backwards. In Britain now a child will wait 2-5 years for diagnosis, and an adult anything up to 10, even with a Dr's referral, unless they are rich and can afford a private consultant. Disgraceful!!!!!

At other times being inside that greenhouse is an extraordinarily sublime and heightened experience of thought and feeling without distraction. In that state of transcendent consciousness some, like Tesla, Van Gogh, Einstein and others found moments of profound clarity in which they uncovered the higher knowledge of arts, sciences and nature that radically changed, enhanced and created the modern world. They were able to **"escape the chains of the ordinary to create the extraordinary" (I. Hale).** Take a step inside and see. The door is open, we are offering you access to our world. We hope you will accept that invitation because Awareness, Acceptance and Appreciation (**The 3 "A"s** – I. Hale) of us as individuals is what we need and what we deserve, not just today, or tomorrow, but every day, that would repay in added social value, many times over.

Our common enemy is ignorance, masking itself as fear. Without human diversity from the norm, cultures would stagnate because progress would be impossible.

Selected Reading and Resources

Aarons, M and Gittens T (1992). The Autistic Continuum: An assessment and Intervention schedule. Nelson BFER.

Attwood, T (1998). Asperger's Syndrome. London. Jessica Kingsley.

Badcock, CR (2009). The Imprinted Brain. Amazon Books.

Baron-Cohen, S (2003). The Essential Difference: Male and Female Brains and The Truth about Autism. Cambridge. Basic Books.

Baron-Cohen, S (1992). Debate and Argument on Modularity and Development in Autism: A reply to Burack. Journal of Child Psychology and Psychiatry. Volume 33, Number 3 pp. 623-629.

Bruce, C (1998). Freefall.
Little, Brown and Company. New York.

David_H_2011_Learning_disabilities_Attention_deficit_Hyperacti vity_Disorder_and_giftedness_Two_case_studies_Gifted_Educatio n_Press_25_3_2_9 https/academemia.edu

The Davidson Institute (2025).
Characteristics and traits of the Gifted Child.
Reno, NV.

Diagnostic and Statistical Manual of Mental Disorders (DSM V). American Psychiatric Association. Arlington, Virginia.

Ehlers, S and Gillberg, C (1993). The Epidemiology of Asperger's Syndrome. Journal of Child Psychology and Psychiatry.

Fitzgerald, M (2003). Autism and Creativity: Is There a Link between Autism in Men and Exceptional Ability? London Routledge.

Fitzgerald, M (2005). The Genesis of Artistic Creativity: Asperger's Syndrome and the Arts. Jessica Kingsley Publisher, London.

Gardner, H (1983). Frames of Mind: The Theory of Multiple Intelligence. New York. Basic Books.

Grandin, T (2008). The Way I See It. Barnes and Noble. New York.

Holick, M F (2011). The Vitamin D Solution. Plume Publishing (Penguin). New York.

ICD-10 (1992). World Health Organization. Geneva: WHO Press.

Kendall, P (2001). Childhood Disorders. Philadelphia. Temple University Press.

Kennedy, A. 2008. Not stupid
Amazon books UK, London.

Kottek, C (1994). 6th Edition: Anthropology: The Exploration of Human Diversity. New York: McGraw Hill.

Kraepelin, E (1927). 9th Edition: Textbook of Psychiatry. Munich. University Press.

Lee, N (Ed) (2019). The Transhumanism Handbook. Switzerland. Springer Nature.

Powell, S, and Jordan R (Ed) (2000). Autism and Learning (A guide to Good Practice). London. David Fulton Publications.

Prakash, V. (2001). A Short Note on the Theory of Multiple Intelligence. Mysore University, India.

Reiss, AL and Dant CC (2003). The behavioral neurogenetics of Fragile X Syndrome analyzing gender brain behavior relationships in child developmental psychopathologies. Volume 15. pp. 927-952.

Reitman, H (2014). Aspertools.
Health Communications Inc. Deerfield Beach, FL.

Remme, W, et al. (2005). Study of Heart Failure Awareness and Personality. European Heart Journal. September 2005.

Ridley, M (2000). Genome. New York. Harper Perennial.

Rostick, E (2006). Male and Female Hormone Testing. Life Extension Magazine. Volume 12 Number 11. November 2006 pp 49-53.

Sanger Institute (2001). The Human Genome Project. Cambridge. Sanger Institute Publications.

Silberman. S Neurotribes (2016) The legacy of autism and how to think smarter about people who think differently (2016) Allen & Unwin. Crows Nest. NSW, Australia.

Schnable, P (2008). Iowa State University. Archives of The Center for Plant Genomics.

Sulston, J (2002). The Common Thread. London: Corgi Book.

Various articles, (2003+).

Venkatesan, S (2004). Children with Developmental Disabilities. New Delhi, Sage Publications.

Vermeer, C (2018). Menaquinone-7 Supplementation Improves Arterial Stiffness in Healthy Postmenopausal Women). Geneva, Switzerland.

Volkmar, F Chawarska, K and Klin, I (2005) Autism in Infancy and Early Childhood Annual Review of Psychology. Volume 56, pp. 315-336.

Wall, K (2004). Autism and Early Years Practice. London: Paul Chapman Publications.

Wilson, R (2003). Special Education Needs in the Early Years. London. Routledge.

Wood, D (1998). 2nd Edition. How children think and learn. Oxford, Blackwell Publishing.

World Health Organization (2006). WHO Archives.

Wurtzel, E (1995). Prozac Nation. New York. Riverhead Books.

Zulkardi, N (1999). CASCADE-MEI Thesis. Enschede: University of Twente Publication.

Seminar and Conference Minutes:

Spiker, D (1999). Seminar. April 1999. Department of Psychiatry and Behavioral Science. Stanford University School of Medicine.

Walton, J (1999). Seminar June 2nd. The art and science of teaching music/dance. Stanford University, Department of Education

Whiteley, P (2004). The Durham Conference Proceedings. Durham University (UK).

Journals:

Journal of the Autism Society of America (ASA). Bethesda, Maryland.

Annals of Dyslexia: Dutch home-based pre-reading intervention with children at familial risk of dyslexia. Sandra G. van Otterloo, Aryan van der Leij. December 2009, Volume 59, Issue 2, pp. 169-195.

Io9. The Lancet Mensa Monthly. National Institutes of Health archives (NIH). Bethesda, Maryland, USA.

Nature Genetics, (2007). February 21 and March 17 Issues.

Psychiatry. jwatch.org. December 10th, 2012. Steven Dubovsky, MD. A predictor for PTSD In deployed soldiers, high pre-deployment CO_2 reactivity was associated with risk for developing PTSD.

Scientific American.

Science 2.0

I. Hale

Credits and Special Thanks

Prof. David P. Burkart (Alembic Enterprises and University of Miami): Artworks, proof-reading, images, and belief.

Prof. Nick Coombs: Support and professional critique.

Ms. Peggy A. Leyva: Support and professional critique.

Mr. Alan Murdoch (University of Birmingham Hospital): Technical consultation.

Ms. Chloe Estelle & Benji: Book cover models.

Chloe Estelle was diagnosed with Asperger's at age 16. The color yellow became a huge part of her life at the same time. Realizing she had more confidence when she wore yellow; she now wears yellow every day. Benji, her superhero service dog, came into her life at age 20. He has allowed her to do things she never thought she could: such as traveling from California to attend college in New York. Chloe began sharing her story as it related to autism and found that it was a more universal tale than she ever thought.

Ms. Annette Lombardi: Photographer for Chloe Estelle.

Annette Lombardi's daughter, Charlie Zuker, diagnosed with Asperger's at 16, is an inspiration and guiding force in her life. Annette loves being surrounded by Asperger adults in her daily life and appreciates the dedication and passions those on the autism spectrum exhibit.

Afterword

When you're diagnosed Autistic, they don't explain to you what autism is. You are given a list of things you struggle with if you can even understand the evaluation that you're handed. I was diagnosed at 16. It was really on me to figure out what that diagnosis meant.

When you start digging into trying to understand autism, you realize it's all written by those who aren't autistic. It's written in a language that is impossible to understand. Criteria often only mentions behavior. I read books and articles and heard podcasts about how I flap my hands, and I don't make eye contact, but I was never given an explanation as to why that felt right.

I stopped looking outside myself and looked within, to others who were autistic. We had conversations. Do you do this? Why do you do this? Books like this ask the questions that help make the struggle easier.

I started being able to communicate. I am unable to process as quickly as others. When a conversation involving multiple people takes place, I need more time to process. In a seminar class, can I send an email that night or the next day with my thoughts. I started to be able to communicate my needs to others.

Autism has nothing to do with behavior. Behavior takes place due to internal processes. I process information entirely differently from the majority of the population. In elementary school we learned bottom-up vs top-down approach to writing essays. Top down: you come up with the thesis first or the main idea. Bottom up: you compile the information first and come up with the thesis or main idea last. Most of the world is set up for top-down thinkers. Autism processing uses bottom up. That wasn't in my evaluation or explained during my diagnosis process. I figured that out on my own. That one simple concept has given me the tools to understand myself.

If I understand my process, then I understand my behaviors. My "rituals" as many professionals called it were part of this process. I had a ritual for everything. I had to jump up and down and run around before brushing my teeth. I had to use a specific toothpaste and toothbrush. When I could communicate what was going on, it no longer was a ritual. I was psyching myself up to do something that was very painful. I had found all the tools to make it the least painful process it could be. Pain receptors often go off during intense sensory activities that don't go off in others. If every time you brushed your teeth you experienced pain, I'm sure your preparation would look ritualistic too.

I was often told to be more flexible. I think I am a very flexible person. I have changed the way I socialize to accommodate everyone else my entire life. I have changed my rituals that help me not experience pain because it bothers other people. I take out my headphones that block out painful noises because it doesn't seem like I am listening. Yet, I'm often met with inflexibility in accepting my needs without explanation.

I could go on and on about how much work I put in so that I can function daily. There is so much put on me to figure it all out. Finding help and support is challenging. Books like this help me understand myself so that I can help myself. Being informed and being informed in a way that helps me understand my own needs—helps me make the choices I need to make to advocate and accommodate myself.

The way this book compiles so much knowledge that took me and others so much time and effort and presents it in an easily digestible format almost makes me sigh in relief that I can refer back to this material over and over instead of scouring for each bit of information. Stories stick with us. I have a hard time taking a fact and knowing how to apply it in real time to my life. Stories give me the ability to see examples of how to use the information as it is shared. Stories take the idea or the hypothetical and make it real. Autistic people are not an idea but real people experiencing life every day.

I am not only autistic, but an advocate for others. I have seen the same story play out myself and with others that I try to help. I also happen to be a twin which has given me a huge individuality complex. It pains me to say that there is a repetitiveness to the autistic experience, but in who we are under the identity or neurotype of autism (validating however you identify), but also the systemic issues. Autism contributes both to the highest highs in my life and the lowest lows. Autism is how I process and see the world and I don't think I would be who I am if I wasn't autistic. This has given me countless opportunities and opened more doors than it has closed. Autism is also a disability with huge challenges and has in fact closed doors that I mourn can never be opened again. These two sides are not in conflict with each other. I wish we could have the good without the bad. You can't change autism, but there are doors I would say could be reopened if people read books like this and made changes to the world. When there is understanding and real change is made to accommodate autism and celebrate the strengths, then my life and so many others could lead a better-quality life with all the opportunities countless others already have available to them.

I had a client point out to me that you surround yourself with certain types of people and experiences based on your job. As an advocate, I am not going to get many people reaching out who are in a great place in life. Most people need an advocate for challenges. I have seen huge challenges every day that no one should ever have to experience. I know that if I took the time to look in my free time (which I try to remember to do just that), there is so much good happening too. I have a spark of hope that people who take the time to read a book like this are working toward that better tomorrow.

Thank you for reading this. Whether you picked up this book for yourself or someone else, I am grateful that you care enough to take in these words and carry them with you even just for a moment. For so long I was silent and not many people tried to listen. Communicating is difficult for me, based on my writing you wouldn't think so. This skill came about by necessity. I would have learned to cook if I did not have access to food at the same age. My missing need was communication. I spent most of my time building this skill in order to meet my needs from a young age. So, thank you for taking in what I have to say.

Chloe Estelle
Autism Advocate

www.ingramcontent.com/pod-product-compliance
Lightning Source LLC
Chambersburg PA
CBHW072227270326
41930CB00010B/2024